THE ULTIMATE GUIDE TO

Energy Healing

The Beginner's Guide to Healing Your Chakras, Aura, and Energy Body

KAT FOWLER

FAIR WINDS

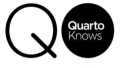

Inspiring | Educating | Creating | Entertaining

Brimming with creative inspiration, how-to projects, and useful information to enrich your everyday life, Quarto Knows is a favorite destination for those pursuing their interests and passions. Visit our site and dig deeper with our books into your area of interest: Quarto Creates, Quarto Cooks, Quarto Homes, Quarto Lives, Quarto Drives, Quarto Explores, Quarto Gifts, or Quarto Kids.

First Published in 2022 by Fair Winds Press, an imprint of The Quarto Group,
100 Cummings Center, Suite 265-D, Beverly, MA 01915, USA.
T (978) 282-9590 F (978) 283-2742 QuartoKnows.com

Fair Winds Press titles are also available at discount for retail, wholesale, promotional, and bulk purchase. For details, contact the Special Sales Manager by email at specialsales@quarto.com or by mail at The Quarto Group, Attn: Special Sales Manager, 100 Cummings Center, Suite 265-D, Beverly, MA 01915, USA.

26 25 24 23 22   1 2 3 4 5

ISBN: 978-0-7603-7175-6

Digital edition published in 2022
eISBN: 978-0-7603-7176-3

Library of Congress Cataloging-in-Publication Data

Fowler, Kat, author.
The ultimate guide to energy healing / Kat Fowler.
ISBN 9780760371756 (trade paperback) | ISBN 9780760371763 (ebook)
1. Energy medicine--Popular works. 2. Self-care, Healtha--Popular works.
LCC RZ421 .F69 2022 (print) | LCC RZ421 (ebook) | DDC 615.8/52--dc23

LCCN 2021029156 (print) | LCCN 2021029157 (ebook)

Design and page layout: Tanya Jacobson, jcbsn.co
Illustration: Mary Ancilla Martinez, @maryancilla.art, www.maryancilla.com

Printed in China

I dedicate this book to each reader who is ready and willing to deepen their spiritual journey into Self-discovery and personal healing. By healing ourselves, we heal the world.

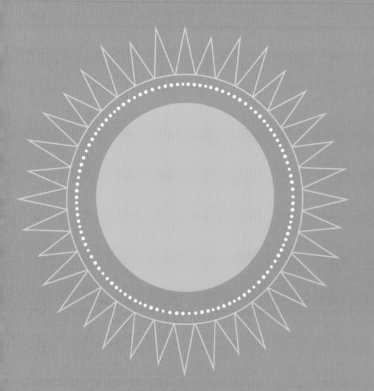

Contents

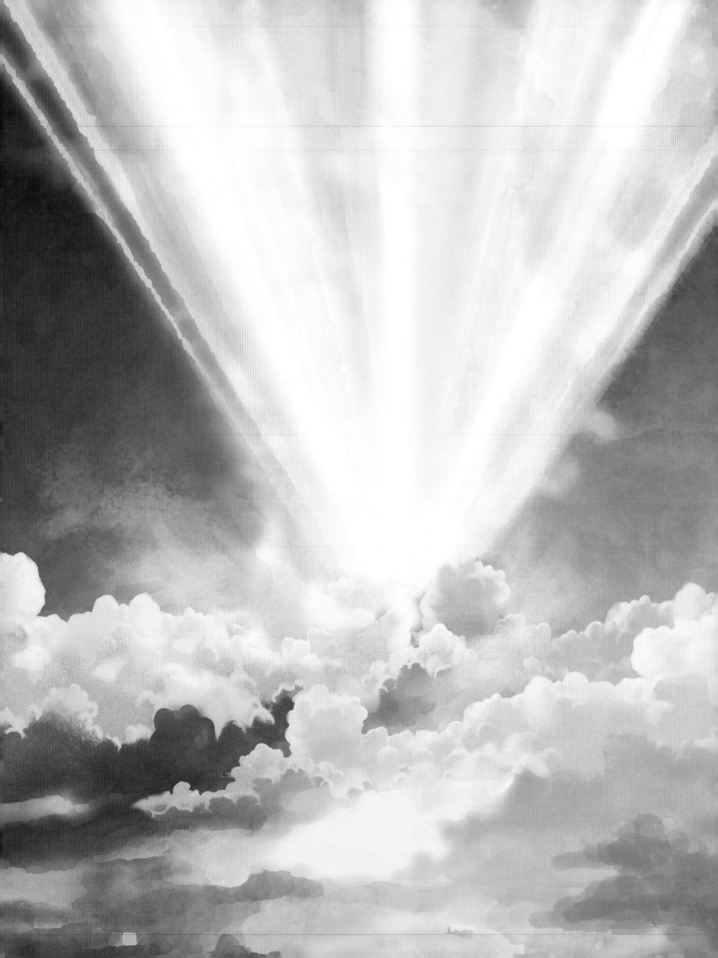

Introduction

Learning to work with your own energy field is where the deepest, most subtle part of your healing begins. Simply setting the intention, and opening yourself up, shows that you are ready and able to practice energy healing. From this first major step on your journey, you can uplevel every part of your life. All things happen in energy first—and this book will guide you on your way.

My personal healing journey began in 2009. I was teaching yoga and meditation, but I still felt like a part of my healing process was missing. Mainstream Western medicine typically takes a "body and mind" approach to healing. Even if it's done holistically, the spiritual and energetic aspects to healing are often kept separate from the physical and psychological—something that is now changing. During my first energy therapy session, what I needed *finally* came to light—it was the third aspect of the triad—spirit.

Energy healing evolved into a beautiful way to learn about myself and who I am. In my first session, I saw visions of my past life as a shaman, where deep healing was needed—I was twenty years old at the time. I had always believed in reincarnation and past lives, being raised in an alternative household. (My fully vegetarian parents met in an ashram.) But I never realized how these things can affect the energy, personality patterns, fears, preferences, and ways we live our lives. I knew this was something special and something I wanted to learn for myself, mainly so I could heal myself and all of these "issues."

Although I was practicing yoga, meditation, and pranayama daily, I now understood there was *so much more* to healing that I never knew existed. I continued to practice and receive energy healing sporadically over the years, along with exploring many forms of holistic healing—acupuncture, working with naturopathic doctors and chiropractors, crystal healing, Chinese medicine, and ayurvedic doctors. For the next decade, I immersed myself in the traditional and ancient yogic spiritual practices and learned multiple forms of energy healing. I also studied the physical body through anatomy, kinesiology, and applied movement and learned how it all relates to our health and well-being.

About a decade later, I had my second massive awakening as my severe childhood trauma of domestic violence and sexual abuse came to the surface, along with several traumatic past lives. It was like hitting the age of thirty unlocked Pandora's box, and the suppressed and stored trauma and emotions of horror and sadness surfaced all at once. I experienced multiple daily panic attacks, agoraphobia, and post-traumatic stress disorder (PTSD). At some of my lowest moments, I could not take the subway or even leave my apartment—everything had to come to a full stop.

I knew my life needed a major change and that what I was going through was a *spiritual* crisis. The work I was doing no longer fulfilled me, and I knew it would take a lot of effort to turn this massive ship around in the right direction. I tried conventional therapy for months, sometimes twice a week, and it was only getting me so far. My therapist recommended I try EMDR (eye movement desensitization and reprocessing), but this had little effect on my early childhood (and past-life) trauma. It was also suggested that I consider taking the Western pharmaceutical route, but I *knew* this was definitely not for me.

Luckily, I could lean on my knowledge of deeper forms of healing, including meditation and energy healing practices. This was my spirit's true path. I began to take it much more seriously: daily meditation became nonnegotiable. Energy healing practices—such as grounding, clearing, and boosting my energy centers and field—became vital parts of my daily routine.

I worked with several energy healers from many lineages and styles, and we turned sessions into one-on-one lessons. I was already channeling energy through my hands and began the transition to practicing advanced energy healing methods. This was tremendously helpful and fascinating to me. I went full-on into my healing process, investing resources and time in taking courses, reading every metaphysical book I could find, and learning new tools and techniques. I could see and feel the powerful effect that each practice was having in my life. Each session I did created more healing for me in an hour than any other path ever had.

In two intense healing years, my panic attacks subsided and my agoraphobia and PTSD were gone. I found a quality of life that was better and more authentic than I have ever lived before. The healing process came with many highs and lows, and there were lots of tears and heart expansions along the way—but I am grateful for every moment, as each brought me closer to my Self.

Energy healing allows you to know yourself in a new way. Everything about you is held within your Akashic Records and in your energy field. The Akashic Records are an energetic library containing the wisdom and knowledge of all time lines, the past, present and future of all beings on Earth, and your personal Soul's journey and evolution. There's absolutely no way to hide from your "stuff" when you begin to heal your energy. It's truly a beautiful process that can move you on the path toward self-love, self-acceptance, and tremendous spiritual growth—if that is your goal. Energy healing and meditation have been the two most powerful tools in my personal healing process. I've lived and experienced it, and continue to expand on it in my own life every day.

This book covers the wide scope of energy healing and meditative practices that I've spent the last decade pouring my life into. I am so honored and joyful that I have this opportunity to share these practices with you. I've infused some of the best practices from many ancient cultures and modern lineages to create a guide for you through your first—or next—steps into energy healing.

While reading this book, you'll gain an understanding of your own personal energy signature and learn to regulate and heal your energy field. My intention is that you receive beautiful energetic upgrades and lightbody activations to help raise your frequency. I hope your connection to your own energy and Soul grows deeper with each new exercise. As you activate the light within you—a light that has been there all along, the light of your true Soul inside—you will see the beauty, innocence, magnificence, and radiance of ALL that you are.

Energy healing reveals so much: You are a beautiful, high-dimensional, high-frequency being of light. You are an individualized spark of the original creative Source, filled with love. You can fully experience your Self on the physical plane of reality now, as a glorious human being at this time. Begin with an open mind and a willingness to heal—from there, there are no limits to how far your journey to self-discovery can go. I wish you love, happiness, and healing as you embark on this new path.

How to Use This Book

Welcome to your personal journey with energy healing. You have consciously decided to begin healing yourself in subtle and profound ways. This is probably not your first time working with healing energy, though it may feel new or unfamiliar. We have been here and incarnated on this Earth many times before and these exercises are an activation of your innate abilities through *remembrance*. Many of us who are attracted to this work now *were* the shamans, healers, and medicine people of the past. We are now stepping back into these roles in big and small ways, becoming the healers of our time.

The training exercises and techniques shared in this book work with the human biofield and come from a variety of traditions, from yogic breathing practices to Native American shaman grounding techniques, along with myriad other practices. It is my hope that this grand collaboration of love, from many benevolent streams of light, flowing through me, into this book, will assist your healing for your highest good.

The book is organized into three parts. The first gives you a foundation of learning about your energetic anatomy, so you firmly understand what you're working with. The second part helps you prepare your energy through meditation, breathing practices, and techniques to allow for the best experience when working with your own energy. The last part of the book guides you through practicing and attuning to energy healing techniques from many traditions and styles of energy healing.

Before starting, dedicate a journal solely to the practices in this book. Take notes about the techniques along the way and include any insights that arise from your experience with each exercise. It'll be amazing to look back in even just one year's time to see how much you have grown.

Please be sure to pace yourself as you move through this book. Each chapter introduces a new level of light and energetic awareness into your field, and your personal healing journey may need time. Follow the exercises in order, as every exercise builds upon the last. You want a solid, strong foundation before moving from one level to the next.

Note: By participating in reading this book, you acknowledge that the information and other content provided, or in any referenced materials, are not intended and should not be construed as medical advice, nor is the information a substitute for professional medical expertise or treatment.

An Opening Meditation

Find a comfortable seat. Allow your spine to be supported and place your feet flat on the floor.

Take a moment to close your eyes. Take a few, slow, easy "sigh" breaths: inhale through the nose and exhale a sigh out through the mouth. Do this two or three times.

Now let your breathing move in and out of the nose and down to the belly. When you inhale, your belly expands. When you exhale, the belly relaxes. Breathe here for a minute, allowing the pace of your breathing to even out. Allow the tension in your body to release with each exhale.

From here, let go of the attention to your breathing and bring your awareness to your heart. Place your hands on your heart and breathe into this region, feeling the warmth and love circulating around this center.

Now set your intentions. You can repeat these out loud or mentally. Take a breath after each one.

I now set the intention through my own effort to use these exercises in this book

to _____ .

- Assist me with healing my own energy.
- Form a loving relationship and communication with my Soul.
- Assist me on my personal organic ascension path.
- Raise my energetic frequency.
- Release all old energies that are no longer serving my highest good.
- Fill every cell and subatomic particle of my being with light and love.
- Activate my Lightbody and upgrade my energetic field.
- Heal, grow, evolve, and integrate all of these changes with ease and grace.

Feel free to add any additional personal intentions made with love at this point.

From here, you can release your hands, relax, and take a few breaths. Notice how shifts are *already occurring* in your energy and field just from setting these powerful intentions.

Be here now, accepting the good that is coming your way. Take as much time as you need. And when you're ready, gently open your eyes.

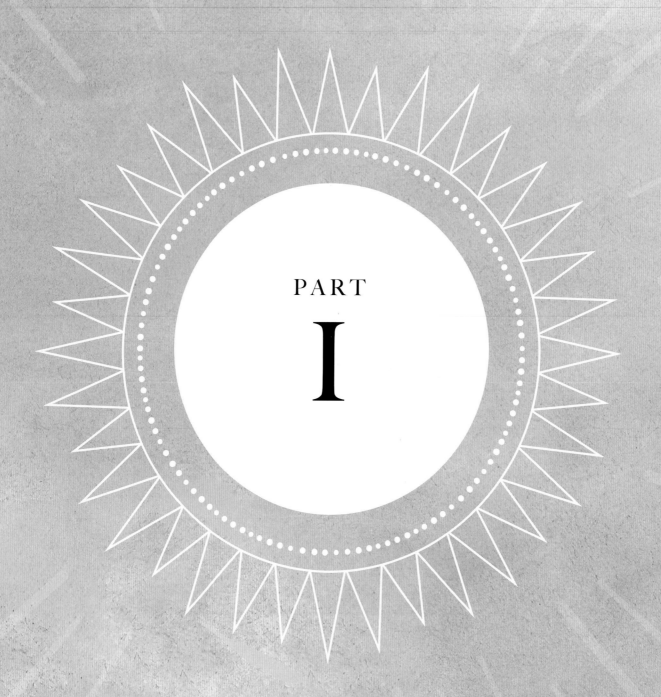

PART

I

GETTING TO KNOW THE BASICS

Energy healing is a subtle art, working with frequencies of a higher vibration than our dense physical reality. In the following chapters, we'll learn about what energy healing is and how it helps us. Then we'll talk about our energetic anatomy—what it looks like and feels like, what it does, and where it's all located—so we'll firmly understand what we're working with. Knowing our own energy signature and how to regulate our field is one of the most powerful tools we can have. It will help us identify and remedy problems, and this will help keep us grounded, centered, and *aligned* within our own being.

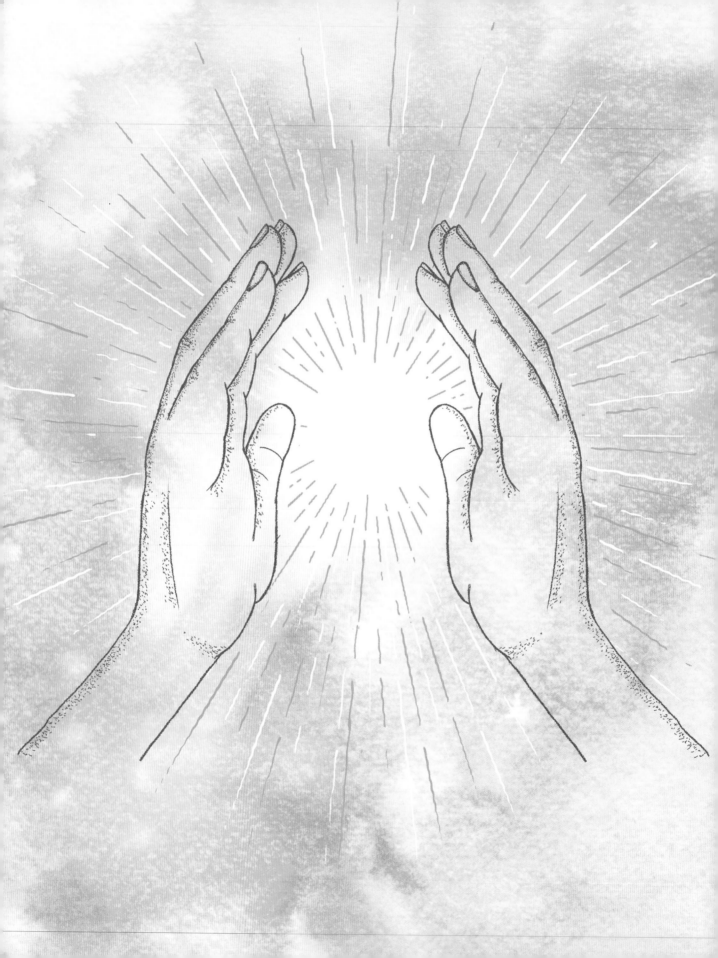

1

What Is Energy Healing?

*E*verything is energy. The physical objects we consider "inanimate," such as rocks, books, or furniture, all hold intelligent light codes of energy that act as the blueprint for their physical existence. Your physical body is comprised of vibrating atoms and subatomic particles of energy, which create the physical form.

Energy healing works with the subtle energy fields and systems in and around the body to create equilibrium and balance. In this chapter, we'll talk about the history and types of energy healing available to you to support your personal spiritual and energetic evolution.

A Brief History of Energy Therapy

The practice of working with energy has been documented since ancient times—some of the first mentions come from around 5000 BCE, from the ancient Hindu texts known as the Vedas. These revered texts speak about the subtle energy in the body, known in the ancient Sanskrit language as *prana*, and discuss various ways to work with it to achieve enlightenment.

The first mention of our energy centers, or the chakras, was around 800 BCE. *Chakra* is also a Sanskrit word meaning "wheel." Energetic practices were also being taught secretly throughout history in places such as Buddhist monasteries, Chinese monasteries, and Indian ashrams; in mystical religions such as Kabbalah and Sufism; in secret Western societies like the Rosicrucians; and in many indigenous cultures throughout the world, where their practices were primarily taught and passed down orally. Many of our modern-day shamanism practices come from ancient medicine men and women who shared their practices through generations.

The traditional Western approach to medicine and healing focuses on the body and the mind. It has them working apart from one another in separate, specialized fields, as opposed to holistically. For complete healing of the individual, we must incorporate the missing factor to the equation—*the spirit*, which is in essence the energy of our being.

But change is finally coming. Recently, the efficacy of Reiki has been studied and incorporated to support cancer patients healing from chemotherapy. Medical intuitives have been utilized in hospitals. Studies of quantum physics have burst onto the scene of mainstream science. Newer technologies and cameras meant to pick up and measure energy signatures and auric fields are now becoming more available. The possibilities for growth are endless.

Paths to Energy Healing

There are many types of energy healing styles; the name itself is really a large umbrella encompassing niche techniques. Many of us have adapted practices, such as acupuncture, Qigong (*qi* being another word for energy), and Reiki (*ki* meaning energy). We also use past-life regression and Akashic Records sessions (reading and healing the Soul and its energetic blueprint). Other practices include Emotional Freedom Technique (also called "tapping"), Intuitive Healing and medical intuition, Pranic Healing, Reconnective Therapy, Quantum Touch, and Theta Healing.

The particular training exercises and techniques shared in this book come from a combination of a different practices, from yogic breathing practices to native shaman grounding techniques, along with many others.

Many people start on this path to seek healing from deep-seated physical or emotional issues. Nothing they've tried has seemed to help—and they've tried everything—and so they open up to the possibility of healing in ways they had not considered before. Others naturally and intuitively gravitate toward working with and reading energy because they already know and have a deep connection to their spirit. Wherever you are in your journey, and whatever path has brought you here, you are in the perfect timing and scenario for your individual Soul.

In energy therapy, we move, release, balance, and heal our energy. As you learn about your own personal energy, and get comfortable with it, you'll begin to understand how and why you operate the way you do. With this baseline, you'll be able to modulate and regulate your energy field on your own. With practice, you can do this to create harmony in your daily experience and interactions in the world.

Through the consistent practice of energy healing, you can:

- Release energetic blocks
- Heal areas in need of repair
- Reestablish the proper flow of energy through the body
- Help release old energy
- Bring balance to the energetic system
- Bring more light into the body to raise your energetic frequency or "vibe"

These are only a few of the possibilities available to you. Energy healing can also bring feelings of deep relaxation and the energy of peace throughout the body. This allows for greater levels of physical, mental, and emotional health and well-being.

There is a process to properly working with energy. One of the first steps is to consistently find a calm place of stillness. Usually this is best found in silence. Sitting in this stillness allows you to sense subtle vibrations and helps you distinguish different frequencies from each other, including what energy is yours and what is not.

As you dive deeper into the metaphysical unseen realms, you will come to understand who you are from the inside out. The saying "energy doesn't lie" is true. Every thought, every powerful emotion, your deepest beliefs, your intentions—it's all held in your energy field. Here are just a few examples:

Repetitive thoughts: These may show up as an etheric form of that object in the aura. For example, you keep wondering when he will finally pop the question, and in your auric field around your head appears a holographic engagement ring—we call these "thought forms."

Stronger emotions: Beyond just being "felt," emotions will appear as color. For example, you head into a meeting after having that big fight with a relative. Even though you're smiling, the emotional layer of your auric field may have an excess of red and certain chakras will show you are actually holding a lot of anger from the experience.

Limiting beliefs: We often place restrictions on our own ability to accomplish things. This can stem from childhood experiences. It may appear as an energy block in the solar plexus chakra.

Everything we do, think, say, and experience is processed and shows up within our energy field. When we embark on the journey of energy healing, we are essentially meeting all aspects of ourselves—the ones from the present moment and those from the past—as energy spans beyond time and space that do not conform solely to third dimensional laws.

Energy healing allows you to access, clear, and heal aspects of yourself that may have been hidden from your awareness for a long time (for some people, potentially their whole lives). It also allows you to create health, balance, and equilibrium throughout your physical body and experience. You can peel off the many layers or "veils" that have hidden or dimmed the light of the true essence that is YOU inside!

How the Energetic Effects the Physical

Before anything occurs physically, there must be the potential for it in the energy field: an idea forms in the energy first and then it moves into a physical stage. For example, when someone "catches a cold," typically the person has been run down energetically for some time, to the point where their aura is weak, open, or has parts missing. Their energetic "defenses" are down and this will lead to or allow pathogens to more easily enter and affect the body.

In Chinese medicine, they call this a Wei Qi deficiency. If the person's energy was very strong and healthy, and their auric field was fortified and full energetically, then that would highly limit the possibility of a cold occurring physically. This is a simplified example, and with health, there are several other energetic factors that can occur that can lead to illness, such as karma and karmic seeds or, occasionally, the person, on a deeper level, taking on an illness for someone else. The cause or reason "why" is not always black and white, but it does always occur first in the energy.

In energy therapy we create shifts quickly on a higher dimensional quantum plane, where time doesn't exist, to which our physical body and environment will then respond. For example, a client comes in with a pain in their neck and shoulders. To balance the energy, first we'll work on releasing energetic blocks or any energetic issues or imbalances in their throat chakra. Then I'll gently open and charge the energy center and areas around it. During the session it's highly likely that they feel a deep sense of peace and potentially some light relief from the issue. Once the energetic "cause" has been removed, it gives their body the natural ability to heal itself as it relaxes. A reduction in pain tends to be a natural side effect of the healing.

Energy healing can only occur when, consciously or subconsciously, the person receiving the healing is ready and willing for a change. And change isn't always easy for most of us. For the healing process to be effective, we must be open to becoming aware of what we've held on to that has created so much disharmony or is no longer serving us. Then, we have to take responsibility for holding on to it and eventually let it go. You can do the work on yourself, but if you are not ready you can only get so far.

Typically, the more acute the issue, the easier it can be to work with or heal, because it hasn't had as much time to become strongly anchored or "physicalized" in the body. The more chronic the issue, the more sessions may be needed for the body itself to make the shifts in the dense physical tissue. Remember, our body is alive and amazing: It is constantly changing and adapting to the information it's receiving. It is always listening to our instructions (our thoughts) in every moment. Miracles, placebo-effect healing, and spontaneous remission occur to those with lifelong issues who are ready to heal in an instant.

Release your preconceived notions when it comes to your potential for healing. Energy healing, just like all healing, happens in layers: we uncover and shed one layer to reveal another, until finally we get down to the center. Additionally, so much of a session's effectiveness comes from setting clear intentions at the start. This directs the energy and tells it where it needs to go. Light energy has its own intelligence, and it will assist your session by moving into exactly the right places in exactly the right amount through setting clear intentions prior to working with it. We'll talk all about the practice of intention setting as we work through the exercises in the book.

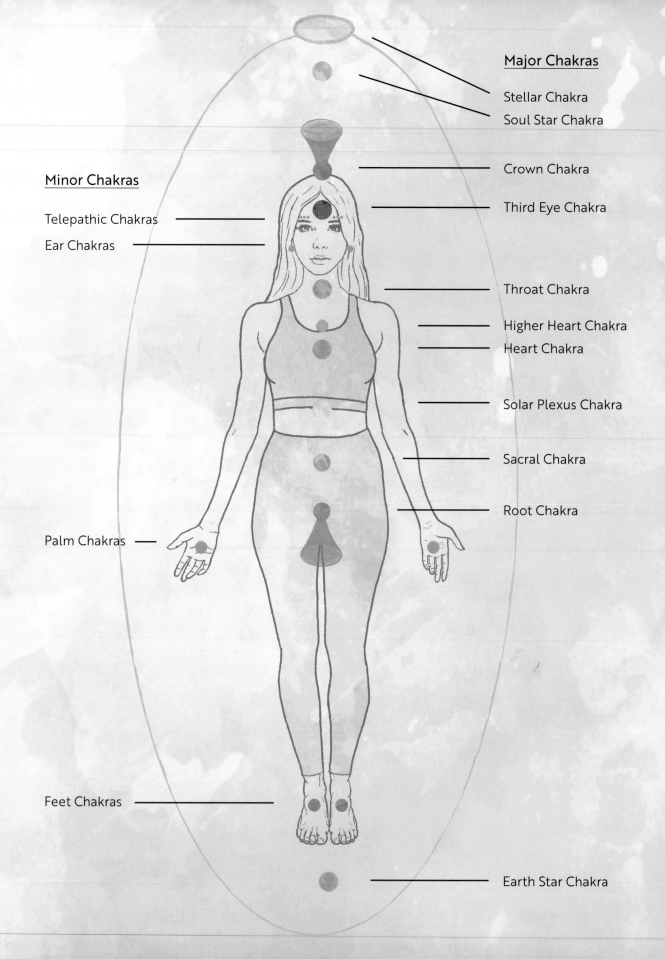

Major Chakras

Stellar Chakra

Soul Star Chakra

Crown Chakra

Third Eye Chakra

Throat Chakra

Higher Heart Chakra

Heart Chakra

Solar Plexus Chakra

Sacral Chakra

Root Chakra

Minor Chakras

Telepathic Chakras

Ear Chakras

Palm Chakras

Feet Chakras

Earth Star Chakra

2

Understanding Your Energetic Anatomy

•

Knowing the fundamental principles of your energetic anatomy will help you tremendously on your journey to healing. In this chapter, we'll talk about the foundational structure of your beautiful body, how your personal lightbody works, and what it looks like. We'll also discuss the different emotional, physiological, and psychological aspects of the energy centers and auric layers that comprise your energetic system. From there, later chapters will help you assess what needs fixing, what needs more fortification, and what needs to come down to create a sound structure.

The Chakras

We are energetic beings of light, here in physical form. We experience this third dimensional physical reality for spiritual growth and Soul evolution. And, as our body grows and develops with us, it responds to the energetic shifts we transmit and receive each day.

The chakras are energy centers located in and extending out of our physical body. These energy centers govern, digest, process, and send out energetic information and signals throughout our physical body. They are essentially the energetic computer command centers that tell our glands, organs, tissues, and body what to do. The chakras fluctuate constantly and adjust according to the energy and patterns of the individual's personality, emotions, habits, thoughts, actions, and lifestyle choices, along with the external stimuli from their environment and relationships.

Within the physical body we have the seven main chakras, which are vortices of light information. They run along the spine and correlate to and regulate the functioning of our glandular endocrine system. We also have several minor chakras and hundreds of tiny chakras all around our body that serve their own separate purposes and functions when it comes to the proper flow of our energy.

Chakras govern the intake and output of energetic electrical signals and photonic light from within and outside of the body. They process everything we experience and how we respond to our environment. This extends beyond the physical and includes how we spiritually perceive and experience the world.

A chakra point looks much like a mini funnel or tornado, with the wider mouth opening facing outward away from the body, and the smaller end of the funnel facing inward. The smaller point intersects our main energetic channel, also called the vertical power current (VPC) or our "ascension column," where the information flows into, meets, and is shared throughout our entire chakra system.

Five of our seven main chakras have a front and a back side to them, while the uppermost and lowest chakra points face upward and downward, respectively. Chakras work interdependently, and are in constant communication with one another. When one chakra is affected, it can affect the overall flow of energy throughout different parts of the body or system.

The Seven Primary Chakras

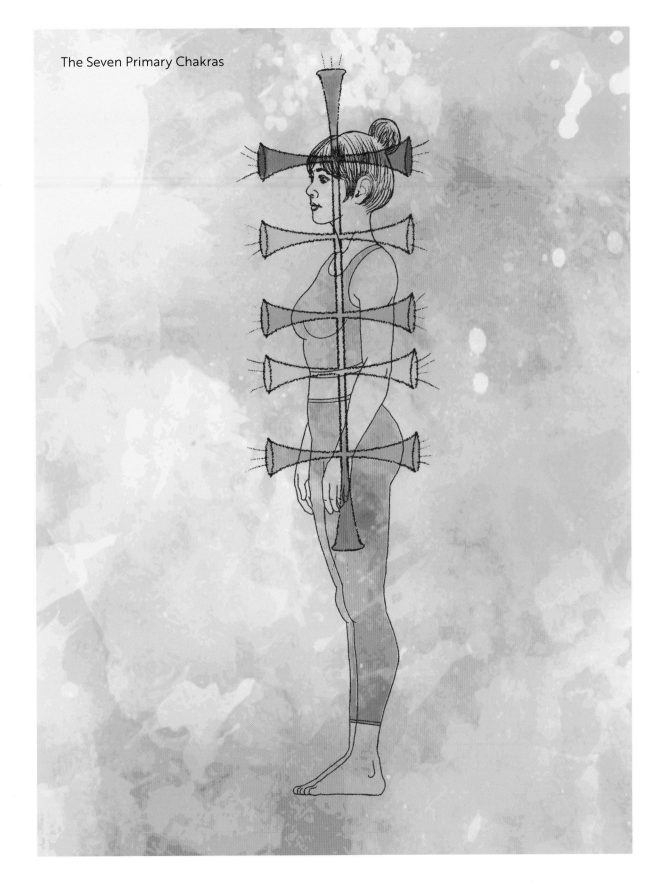

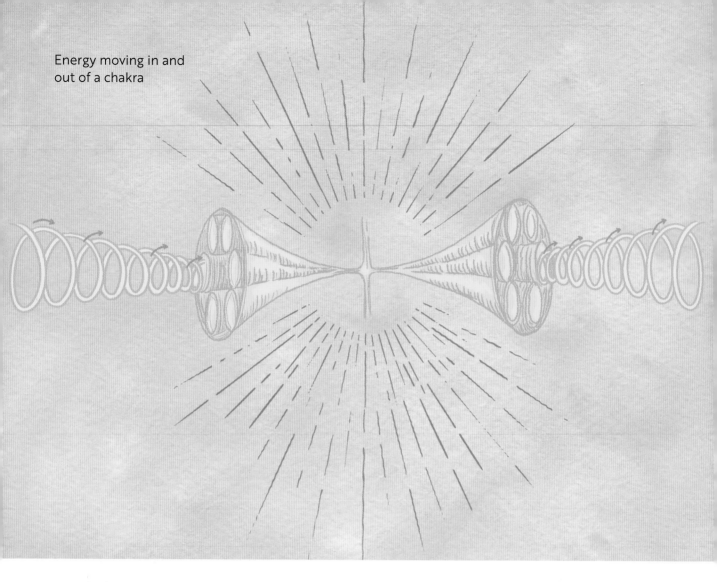
Energy moving in and out of a chakra

The chakra system functions on energetic color frequencies, moving from the deeper, slower, grounded, red root chakra upward to the vibrant violet color of the crown. The range is similar to the way sound waves operate: from low and slow to high and fast. Each chakra has its own characteristic information that it handles and processes, and lessons to learn and master to activate and open, or "unlock," the energy center. The chakras are constantly oscillating and adjusting according to the information being transmitted or received. The outer openings of the chakras dilate open and closed, similar to a lotus flower or the pupil in our eye. The speed of the "spin" or rotation of the chakra will vary according to the amplitude of energy moving in or out of it at the time. For example, a singer performing on stage usually has a throat chakra dilated wide open, spinning fast. A swami or monk, living in silence, and spending most of their time in meditation, would have a throat chakra that is minutely dilated and spinning at a slower rate.

Ways the Chakras Affect the Body

The seven main chakras are energetically associated with the endocrine system: each individual chakra manages the energy of each individual endocrine gland. The chakras also affect the entire region of the physical body, including internal organs, bones, muscles, and tissues, that they are in line with.

Working with or viewing a chakra gives us good insight into a person's state of wellness, physically, mentally, emotionally, and spiritually. Having the proper flow of energy in an area is what can create health and healing in the body, or, conversely, pain and stagnation. When a chakra is operating in a healthy way, we usually find that the correlating area is healthy, and the same is true in reverse. Someone with chronic back pain, for example, is likely having some issue with the chakra in that region.

Consistently reading your own energy field will provide you with invaluable feedback into your own inner workings and where you could use some healing and strength in your life. A healthy chakra can filter and allow the proper information into and out of your system and translate it into the proper discernable messages. When in balance, your chakras can instantaneously adjust to the flow, rhythm, and speed of the information. It can also modulate it so you are only receiving as much as you can physically handle in each moment.

If there is an excess of energy flowing into or out of the chakra, we may find chaotic signals, swelling, nerve issues, anxiety, and many other imbalances. If there is a lack of energy flowing through the center, then we may find we have pain or cramping, degeneration, or different sorts of health issues. The glands tend to be directly affected by this, and just one gland not functioning optimally—for example, the pituitary, or "master gland," which regulates the hormonal system—can wreak havoc throughout the entire physical body. An unhealthy chakra, which may be depleted, damaged, blocked, or blown open due to trauma or drug use, can no longer properly take in, send out, or compute the energetic information. It may misinterpret or distort the information, or the translation into the body may be indecipherable.

The amount of time that a chakra has consistently been in an unhealthy state, along with the severity of the imbalances, will determine the level of the physical, mental, emotional, and spiritual imbalance that is occurring. The chakras can affect one issue, a combination, or all of them, depending on the reason why the original energetic issue occurred.

A healthy chakra's resting dilation level is different for everyone. For example, on a scale of 1 to 100, a healthy root chakra may be dilated open 20 percent for one individual according to their needs. For another, this may feel like it's too closed and uncomfortable; their typical healthy resting dilation may be around 60 percent. Modulating your chakras—even above or below the healthy range of 15 to 85 percent—can be used to address healing.

For example, someone may find being on Earth too harsh due to the energetic imprint of childhood trauma. Sensitivity to these imprints makes it uncomfortable to stay put and be grounded within their physical body, and they often daydream and energetically "leaves their body" through their 100 percent dilated crown chakra. Their wide-open crown chakra was a coping mechanism and method of "escape" from dealing with the traumas of the past that are stored within the physical body. Their lower chakras store the past traumas, and they are practically closed and avoided. This compounds their extreme difficulty with grounding.

Signs of Imbalances

Chakras can become blocked or imbalanced for a multitude of reasons. These include:

- Traumatic events from this life or a past life
- Drug use, specifically mind-altering psychoactive drugs (including plant medicines)
- Chronic environmental stressors
- Consumption of unhealthy inorganic foods
- Inorganic substances
- Codependent relationship patterns, which can create things such as energy cords and hooks
- Consistent negative thoughts or moods
- Old programming or belief systems

There are *many* other ways and reasons that chakras can become blocked. What matters is identifying the imbalance, and then clearing, releasing, and rebalancing the flow of energy within them.

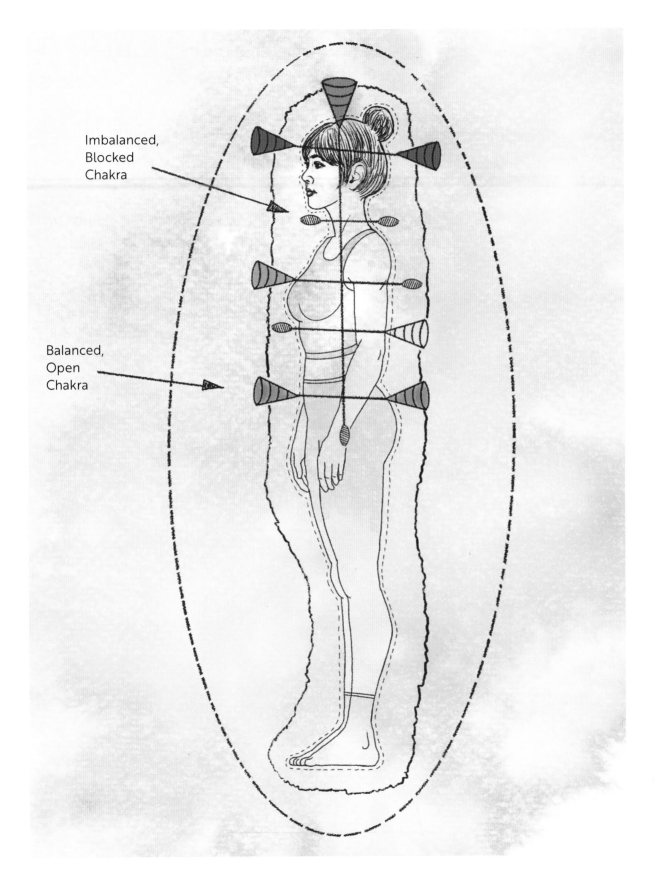

Imbalanced,
Blocked
Chakra

Balanced,
Open
Chakra

Through self-discovery about their energetic patterns, this person can clear and heal these energetic blocks and begin grounding regularly. In a remedial healing way, they can also dilate their crown chakra down to 5 to 10 percent to prevent being "up in the clouds," while simultaneously dilating open their root and lower chakras to help maintain a grounded connection with the earth. Through extensive practice and conscious effort, the chakras can be regulated and naturally hold these energetic patterns. After a few months, this person will be able to stay in their body, while still experiencing the higher spiritual planes of existence—all while maintaining stability and health throughout their system. These changes create stability, health, growth, and a sense of groundedness in their daily living, and they'll find the balance of both worlds within themself.

Consciously understanding your energetic anatomy and patterns, and then using the knowledge to heal and remedy those imbalances, can have a tremendously beneficial effect on your entire life, in all areas. I have experienced this myself, as have a large majority of spiritual seekers (and starseeds).

When a chakra is blocked or imbalanced, you may feel or sense that something is "off." Depending on the severity of the imbalance, this can manifest as feeling emotionally, creatively, or intuitively stunted. In more severe cases, it may manifest as physical pain, anxiety, depression, sleep disorders, and health issues. Usually, the quicker we can identify an issue and remedy it with energy healing and healthy physical habits, the higher our chances of success!

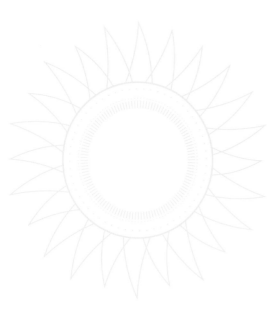

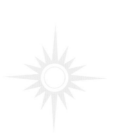

We've become so used to living with unhealed trauma and constant stress that many of us don't know what it's like to feel energetically aligned. One of the best ways to learn to intuitively spot an imbalance is to take an honest assessment of all areas in your life: physical, relational, mental, emotional, and spiritual. Do this *without* any judgment, but simply as a neutral observer. Finding and maintaining neutrality in your practice can create the awareness needed to continuously move forward on the path to your own personal healing with ease and grace.

Soon you'll be able to catch when something feels off *immediately*. Then you can work to clear, release, and rebalance your energy. With dedication and practice, you can understand your own energy signature, and what it feels like when it's healthy, vibrant, and stable. This self-knowledge allows you to become your own best healer on your personal spiritual journey to freedom.

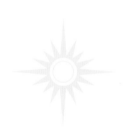

The Seven Main Chakras

We categorize chakras into three main groups. They are interdependent, in that "higher" does not necessarily mean "better." We need ALL of our chakras to be healthy and functioning to achieve health and balance in our lives, and to help us move forward on our spiritual evolutionary paths.

The lower chakras: the root, sacral, and solar plexus chakras
The lower chakras address our earlier earthly lessons dealing with survival, physical health, our relationships, and our will. These all mainly work with regulating our experiences within the physical realm.

The bridge or middle chakra: the heart chakra
The chakra in the middle, the heart chakra, is literally the energetic bridge between the physical and the metaphysical realms, the bridge between the gross and the subtle experiences.

The upper chakras: the throat, third eye, and crown chakras
The upper chakras mainly concern the spiritual realms and higher lessons of learning.

Patterns form in the energy according to an individual's level of consciousness and level of healing. Here are a few examples:

- The lower chakras are open but upper chakras are closed: The person may feel like they are operating on autopilot and cut off from their spirituality.

- The upper chakras are open but the lower chakras are closed: The person may feel completely ungrounded, airy, spaced out, and may have trouble operating in daily living.

- All or most of the chakras are consistently small, slow, or depleted: The person may be very "low energy," fatigued, or depressed.

- All or most of the chakras are too open, too fast, or overcharged: The person may have problems with concentration, nervous disorders, and mental health issues due to overstimulation.

- The energy flow needs to be "just right" to maintain balanced physical, mental, and emotional well-being. Ideally, we would like all the chakras to be open and spinning properly; dilated to a unique healthy percentage for the individual; and balanced and in harmony with the system, as opposed to top- or bottom-heavy.

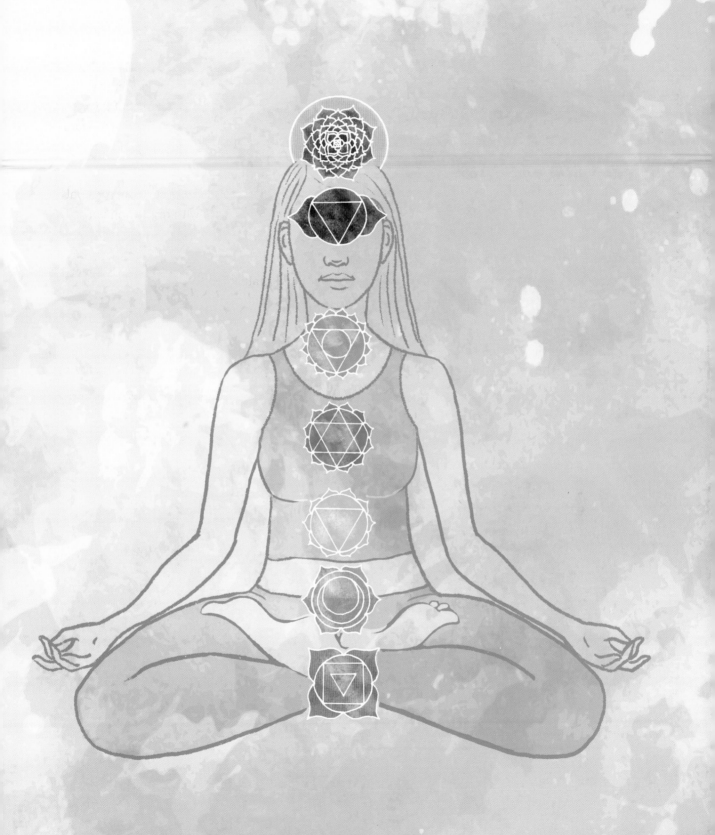

The Root Chakra

Location: Base of the pelvis, around the perineum and close to the tailbone

Color: Beautiful red

Sanskrit name: Muladhara

Associated gland: The adrenals

Energy and lesson: Survival and moving out of fear

The root chakra governs our physical health and vitality, our ability to manifest and maintain abundance (or lack thereof), and our ability to take care of ourselves stably. It can also deal with past-life issues.

When the root chakra is in balance, we feel *secure, safe, and stable*, are physically in good health, have lots of physical energy, are flowing with abundance, and are living comfortably with our ability to take care of ourselves.

When the root chakra is out of balance, we can have unreasonable and consistent fears, feel "unsafe" or fatigued, and have a strong identification with victim consciousness, where for whatever reason outside of ourselves (and there will always be such a reason), we consistently struggle with taking care of our shelter, life, and survival. It may also signal financial issues.

An excessive, or overcharged, root chakra will lead us to strong states of anger or aggression, a highly materialistic focus on money and greed, and a need to control and dominate everything around us. A depleted, or undercharged, root chakra will lead to excessive fear and insecurity.

Our root chakra is also one of the best ways to energetically "root down" and connect with the high-vibrational core of Mother Earth. Earth energy is so nourishing and healing to the root chakra, and our ability to ground and connect with the Earth is a key factor in maintaining a stable, even-keeled emotional state and vibrant physical health.

We're spiritual beings living in a physical body here on planet Earth, and even though this book is all about energy healing, we do need to deeply honor and respect our physical vessels in this lifetime, as they *are a part of the Earth herself*. We will discuss much more about the benefits of grounding and making the energetic connection with the higher dimensional aspects of the inner Earth, but for now just remember the root chakra's important role and connection to our ability to connect with Gaia.

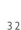

The Sacral Chakra

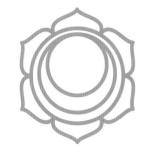

Location: Above the root chakra, below the navel

Color: Vibrant orange

Sanskrit name: Svadhisthana

Associated gland: Ovaries and testes

Energy and lesson: Interpersonal relations and healthy sexual expression

Our sacral chakra has everything to do with our emotions around situations and relationships with others, including our ability to healthily, sensually experience and express our sexuality. This is also a primary center when it comes to our creative energy.

When the sacral chakra is in balance, we feel harmonious in our relationships with others, and very comfortable with our divine sexual energy: our sexual organs are healthy, and we feel a sense of vibrancy and vitality in our lives.

When the sacral chakra is imbalanced, we can feel lonely, isolated, or jealous; have health issues with the sexual organs; and have major repression or fears around expressing our sexuality. When the sacral chakra is depleted, we may feel like we have almost no libido, lack the drive to connect with others, or experience impotence. When the sacral chakra is excessive, we may unconsciously be misusing, exchanging, or giving away our sexual energy to anyone who will give us attention, and we may have many issues with the relationships in our lives.

The Solar Plexus Chakra

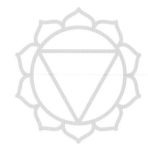

Location: Below the rib cage and above the navel

Color: Golden yellow like the sun

Sanskrit name: Manipura

Associated gland: Pancreas

Energy and lesson: Developing and consciously asserting our self-confidence, will, and personal power in this world as conscious creators

The solar plexus chakra has everything to do with how the body digests and metabolizes substances and information. When the solar plexus is healthy and in balance, we feel a healthy dose of confidence and are not afraid to be who we are; we feel empowered and respect ourselves and others deeply. We even carry a sense of joy in our daily lives.

When the solar plexus is out of balance, we may feel afraid to decide and stand up for ourselves, or on the other end of the spectrum, are constantly engaged in power struggles in different areas of our lives. When this chakra is out of balance, we may energetically "feel a pit in our stomach" and even have digestive issues of all sorts. We also may aggressively bully or try to impose our will on others.

Having a healthy balanced solar plexus chakra allows us to move into a creator state, where we are healthily asserting our will in our reality, while respecting boundaries and manifesting and creating positive changes in our lives. We are empowered and feel like we can take on anything that comes our way!

The Heart Chakra

Location: Center of the chest

Color: Emerald green, and additionally pink

Sanskrit name: Anahata

Associated gland: Thymus

Energy and lesson: Unconditional love, compassion, vulnerability, and forgiveness

The heart chakra concerns our ability to express, give, and receive the energy of love. When the heart chakra is in balance, it's easy to give and receive love and have compassion for *all* beings—not just our family or small circles, and not just humans.

When the heart chakra is out of balance, we can feel closed off emotionally, and we are uncomfortable giving or receiving the energy of love from others, or even ourselves. We may hold grudges and resentment against others, and have fears of feeling unsupported or hold the false belief that we are unlovable at a deep level. This tends to be a core wound of many old Souls (which many of you reading this book are) that has developed over many lifetimes of being a spiritual, sensitive, and awakened Soul in the darker ages of time. Learning to release these conditioned fears and beliefs, and release the resentment and hatred in our hearts, lets love flow in and through and creates harmony in the heart chakra.

When the heart chakra is depleted, we may feel closed off to the possibility of love in any form; when it's in excess, we don't have healthy boundaries around giving and receiving and when it's appropriate to express the energy of love. When there is an imbalance, we may experience physical issues around the heart, lungs, upper spine, shoulder blades, arms, or circulation. When it is in balance, we feel ease in our ability to give and receive love in our relationships, including with ourselves.

Ah, the Heart Chakra

The heart chakra is one of the most important chakras for creating and maintaining love and harmony in our lives. In ancient yogic texts that speak about enlightenment, we learn that this occurs through raising the energy up through each open and balanced energy center, one by one, from root to crown, to achieve oneness with God, bliss, and a merging with the Universe. This is true, and if your goal is enlightenment, then that is the process and way to go. In the past, this was achieved through intense renunciation and meditative practices, by many Mahatmas, swamis, and monks. However, if you're looking to achieve these states, while still being in touch with society, family, friends, humanity, and the world around you, then after mastering the lessons of all seven chakras, move your awareness back into your heart chakra.

The symbol for this chakra is two interlocking triangles, one pointing upward, representing the energy of the lower chakras moving upward, and one pointing downward, representing the energy of the upper spiritual centers moving downward, where they both meet, merge, and *integrate* in the heart, symbolizing balance and harmony within the entire system. The heart chakra is like a portal, or stargate, into all higher states of consciousness, while staying grounded *within* the physical body, meaning you remember everything and are conscious of it; you don't energetically vacate the body to have these higher experiences, you have these higher experiences *within*.

The energy of the heart chakra is love and is the storehouse of our supreme Soul energy. It is where we go when we want to meet the God *inside*. When operating from the heart chakra in our daily living (after we have integrated all the lessons from all seven chakras), everything becomes naturally infused with the energy of love. We can feel the energy of unity and love for all beings in the most cosmic and grounded way.

The energy of the heart chakra is all about unconditional love and compassion—not necessarily empathy, as compassion and empathy are two distinctly different qualities. When we speak of love, we mean divine love, the love that is so pure and so strong that it overpowers and outshines all other emotions. It is beautiful, truthful, strong, stable, and supportive. It is *not* the unstable version of romantic love. This is a divine, never-ending, nonjudgmental, unconditional, beautiful love, that if experienced for even a moment would make you weep. It is the pure innocent energy of the divine presence of God (Source, the Universe, a higher power, whatever you'd like to call it) that is shining through in this energy.

The Throat Chakra

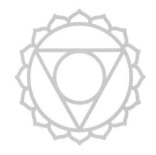

Location: Center of the neck

Color: Sky blue

Sanskrit name: Vishuddha

Associated gland: Thyroid

Energy and lesson: Conscious, clear communication and sharing our deepest spiritual truth

When the throat chakra is healthy, communication is easy and flowing, but when there is an imbalance, we may have speech issues, lose our voice, be afraid to speak up for what we believe in, or have physical issues in the above areas. When it is out of balance, there is also a tendency toward gossiping, lying, or being untruthful with our word.

I have seen many old Soul lightworkers struggle with this area, coming from many past lives in an older energy where we were persecuted for speaking about spirituality or sharing our spiritual gifts. The throat chakra, when consciously healed and activated, allows us to express our highest divinity in the physical world through sound, speech, writing, light language, and song.

The Third Eye Chakra

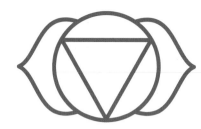

Location: Between the eyebrows

Color: Indigo

Sanskrit name: Ajna

Associated gland: Pituitary

Energy and lesson: Seeing reality clearly and truthfully

The third eye chakra is the center where the ego is met and challenged and must ultimately be balanced to release the lower personality perceptions (illusions) and see the world through the divine lens (that of our higher self) of truth. This is where we see and learn information that is relative to the evolution of our Soul, and the main lesson is seeing past all illusions: personal, societal, religious, and cultural. When this occurs, our clair gifts activate: the gift of clairvoyance, or "clear seeing," the gift of clairaudience, or "clear hearing," and many more. These are our extrasensory gifts. This chakra (like most other chakras) can be damaged or closed down by experiencing childhood trauma, seeing traumatic events, having fear around what we may see beyond the veil, or doubts about our own abilities.

When the third eye is balanced, we see the truth in all situations. We feel and think clearly and trust what we see and believe. When it is out of balance, we have a strong tie with our ego, we push away the truths and lessons that may benefit us spiritually, we get into mental loops and play out false scenarios and fights in our heads, and we don't want to "see" the things about ourselves that can help us grow. This also may manifest physically as eye issues, migraines and headaches, brain issues, and endocrine imbalances. In excess, we may have no boundaries or control around what we see beyond the veil, as we may view things that are harmful to us psychologically, or pry and prod into other people's business intentionally and without permission. Ultimately, when the third eye is consciously activated, we have a stable mind and see the truth within all situations.

The Crown Chakra

Location: Top of the head

Color: Ultraviolet

Sanskrit name: Sahasrara

Associated gland: Pineal (melatonin levels, ability to regulate our sleep)

Energy and lesson: Spiritual connection to a higher power and beliefs

This chakra is our pure connection to oneness, divinity, or pure consciousness. This is our connection to all that is. It commonly gets shut down through dogmatic religious or familial programming around what we "should" believe spiritually, or around the fear of a "punishing" God. When the spiritual energy of this chakra has been awakened, we achieve a state of enlightenment, bliss, nirvana.

When we have mastered the lessons of this chakra, we have a free-flowing, fully conscious connection with the Divine. It is us and we are it; there *is no* separation. When this chakra is out of balance, we may feel cut off from our spiritual connection and have a lot of doubt in our beliefs around spirituality and our ability to connect with a higher power. When it's in excess, we may engage in escapism or an addiction to spirituality to the point where daily living in the physical realm is neglected. A healthy, balanced, and open crown chakra allows us to send and receive the divine cosmic inspiration and messages available to us, through practices like stillness and meditation.

By now, just from reading about the chakras you may already have a strong idea as to where the health of your chakras and the imbalances may lie. The more you know, the easier it is for you to identify your patterns and work to heal the energy around them so you can live a calm, centered, and happy life.

The Minor Chakras

Our minor chakras range from the size of a pea to expand to about the width of a golf ball. They function similarly as transmitters and receivers of energetic information in the body. Separately, each meridian point in the body used in traditional Chinese medicine is also a microscopic chakra point. The following are the principal minor chakras we will use in our practices. There are additional minor chakras, including behind the knees, in the elbows, behind the shoulder blades (where the appearance of "angel wings" can occur from when activated with love), above the third eye, and around the crown.

The Feet Chakras

The feet chakras are smaller chakras on the soles of our feet, pointing downward away from the body, similar to the root chakra. These chakras connect us with the Earth, keep us rooted, and help us move forward with our plans in life. When these are blocked, we may have trouble grounding, connecting with nature, or energetically "putting our foot down" when it comes to our plans in life. The feet chakras connect to our leg meridians and help run the energy up into and down out of our root chakra when working with channeling and moving energy.

The Palm Chakras

The palm chakras are smaller chakras in the middle of our palms. They concern creatively putting out our energy into the world, and our ability to give and receive energy. These chakras need to be activated to perform hands-on healing. Energetically, it is universally believed that our left side represents our divine feminine aspects, and our right side represents our divine masculine aspects. This is true for our physical body and for our energy. The feminine energy has to deal with receiving and the masculine energy is about giving. When it comes to using our palm chakras, they can both take in and send out healing energy, but it is typically much easier to receive energies with the left hand and to give energies with the right hand. I do believe this is also why the majority of the population is naturally right-handed. When the palms are facing up, we tend to be receiving; when the palms are facing down, we are grounding energy (though there are always exceptions). The palm chakras are connected to the arm meridians, which are connected to the throat and heart chakras. There are different techniques for drawing in, working with, and sending out energy through the hands that we will discuss in depth in later chapters.

The Telepathic Chakras

There are several telepathic chakras that allow for the gift of telepathy to occur. There are two main telepathic chakras, one on each temple, and then there are several much smaller ones located right above the eyebrows and move down the side of the face toward the ears, similarly to eyeglasses frames. When these are too open, we can hear thoughts and conversations and inappropriate things from others without control; this can also lead to serious headaches around that region. When they are in balance, we can think clearly without external interruption, meditate with ease, and receive messages from our spirit guides and higher self when needed.

The Ear Chakras

The ear chakras activate the gift of clairaudience, and when open allow us to hear clear messages from the Divine. When this gift is activated, you will literally hear your guides as clear as day like you would hear a person standing next to you. When it's overactive or damaged, you may be hearing random voices with no control, or you hear nothing at all when it comes to speaking with your guides or receiving information while meditating. These centers concern hearing divine and spiritual information from higher dimensional guides and beings of light.

The Transpersonal and Subpersonal Chakras

The transpersonal and subpersonal chakras are spiritual centers of a higher dimensional frequency than our main seven chakras and minor chakras. They rarely reside within the physical body. The ones listed tend to reside between the eighth and twelfth dimension. There are more levels of chakras than those that are listed, spanning within, above, and beyond the twelfth dimension, but for now we'll discuss the main chakras that you may be working with throughout this book.

The Earth Star Chakra

The earth star chakra is a subpersonal chakra in the shape of an orb located about two feet below our feet; it grounds and holds our higher dimensional blueprint for our Soul's plan here on Earth. This is the color of platinum. When activated, we can ground and connect with Gaia almost instantaneously. Our grounding connection will feel much stronger and the frequency of the Earth energy coming in can flow in greater amounts. The earth star becoming activated has a lot to do with us moving onto our higher time lines and path of divine service.

The Higher Heart Chakra

The higher heart chakra, or thymus chakra, has to do with universal love and acceptance. It is the only exception to the transpersonal chakras, as it's in the physical body (at the thymus) and has vortices in the front and back of the body. This chakra's color is aqua and, when activated, allows energetically for etheric DNA recoding and healing, Soul level healing, and access to our innate Akashic Records within our DNA. The three energies of the higher heart chakra, including the main heart chakra and the energy around and within the physical heart organ (also called the "sacred heart"), when combined and activated, are a portal into the higher dimensions, where only pure love and oneness exist.

The Soul Star Chakra

The soul star chakra holds the majority of the energy of our Soul's light within it. The journey to activating the soul star is through meditation—simply breathing with intention, gently bringing in more and more of the light codes (little packets of information, similar to a zip file) that contain your original Soul light. We do have the energy of our Soul within the body, but typically only a small percentage. Once we purify the body through healthy eating and living and detoxification practices and meditation, then we can literally hold more of our light within our physical vessel. When activated, we are on our mission and are merging and connecting with our Soul's light now within the body. We may have started at holding 10 percent of our Soul's light in the body before awakening, but after conscious intentional energy healing we can hold energies of up to 80 percent of our Soul's frequency within the body. When one can hold 100 percent, they have achieved ascended mastery, like Jesus Christ or Buddha did, who were living as "en-light-ened" masters walking the physical Earth plane. The color of this chakra orb is a beautiful gem-quality magenta.

The Stellar Chakra

The stellar chakra is the twelfth dimensional chakra portal that exists two to three feet above our heads. This is in the shape of a disk, and I believe is what has been typically depicted when it comes to the ascended masters and angels with halos around their heads. This is like a cosmic receiver of very high-dimensional frequencies from places like the galactic center, our sun and the grand central sun, and from our highest Soul core group, or our monadic presence, which allows us to bring more light into our energy field and lightbody. This is the beautiful color of shimmering gold. When we work with the frequency of gold, we are pulling it in from this place. There are several techniques to activate this chakra to bring in the beautiful, protective, and strengthening frequency of gold to assist our energy practices. Having this color around you also allows your higher self and angels to more easily work with you.

The Aura

Our aura is an energetic bubble that exists all around the body and extends outward, in layers, three to five feet wide in all directions. Each layer of the aura contains a new set or grouping of information within it, in a new dimensional field of existence.

A healthy aura has the shape of a balloon or a well-rounded egg. When our aura is depleted or damaged, it can be misshaped, missing areas, or have tears in its matrix. When this occurs, we have the potential of leaking our energy out, forming unhealthy cords with others, or not having the proper filters necessary when it comes to the incoming information around us.

Our auras, just like our chakras, are constantly changing and adapting according to our inner perceptions and outer reality shifts. Our aura expands when we're happy and joyful and contracts when we're sad and fearful. An expanded, full aura is infinitely superior in protection over a weak, depleted, small aura with a light shield around it.

Having a strong, healthy, full aura is our best line of energetic protection above all other techniques. The emotion of love is one of the strongest tools for boosting our auric field. Our aura also becomes vibrant through simple practices. These include:

- Meditation
- Breathwork
- Getting natural sunlight
- Eating organic foods
- Sleeping well
- Exercising
- Connecting with nature
- Keeping your thoughts and vibrations high

When our aura is weak, we are more prone to physical illness and unconsciously uninvited energetic intrusions by external energies into our field. The following all individually and collectively contribute to an unhealthy aura:

- Low-vibrational music and words
- Heavier emotions
- Prolonged stress
- Stored trauma
- Inorganic foods and inorganic substances
- Excessive use of technology
- Exposure to electric and magnetic fields (EMFs)
- Poor sleep
- Sedentary lifestyle
- Alcohol and drug use
- Disconnection from nature

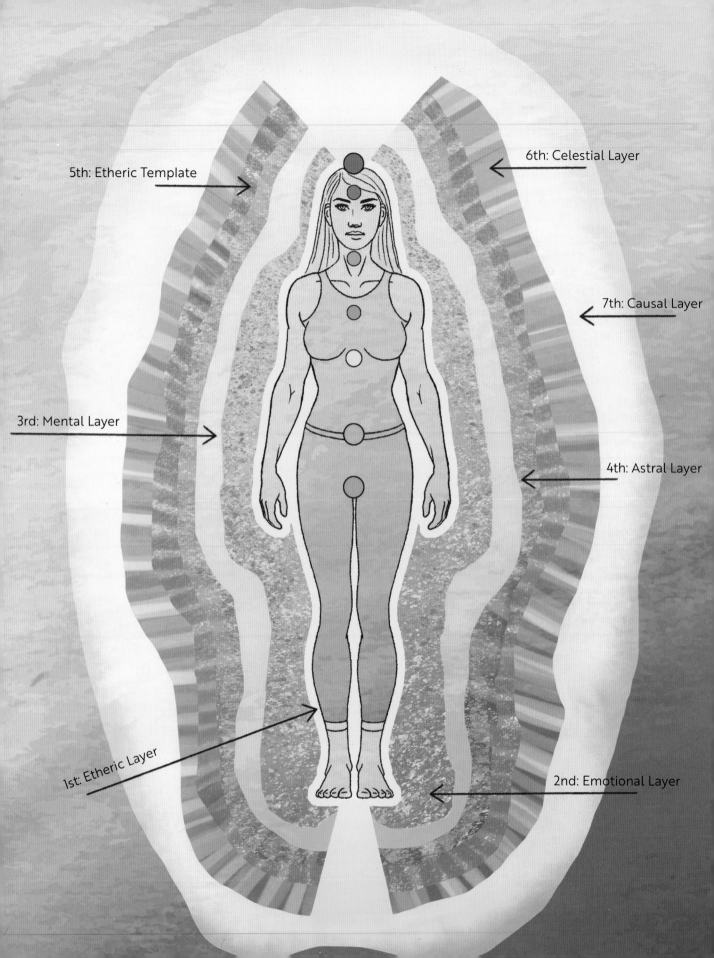

5th: Etheric Template

6th: Celestial Layer

7th: Causal Layer

3rd: Mental Layer

4th: Astral Layer

1st: Etheric Layer

2nd: Emotional Layer

The health of our energy *depends on us* and our conscious decisions around what we consume and continuously expose ourselves to, along with our practice of meditation and sitting in stillness. We *absolutely* have the power to regulate, heal, and strengthen our auric field now that we know what it takes.

The Seven Layers of the Auric Field

When speaking in energetic terms, as multidimensional human beings, we exist in many dimensions all at once: we have aspects of Self in a large range of dimensional frequencies. The seven layers of the auric field move up in dimensional frequency: the slowest, or most dense layer, is closest to the physical body. The fastest, or most subtle layer, is furthest away from the physical body. The first field correlates with the first dimension, the second field with the second dimension, and so on.

Similar to the chakras, the first three layers of the auric field have a lot to do with our physical reality and how the physical body and lower personality self perceives and relates to our experiences and the world around us. The fourth layer corresponds to the heart chakra and likewise is the astral bridge, or the connecting realm between the physical and spiritual. The upper three layers concern how our spirit feels and experiences the reality we live in.

First: The Etheric Layer

Location: Wraps all around the skin
Correlations: Our physical experience, physical health, and wellness
Chakra: Root

When healthy, this layer tends to appear and remain a beautiful vibrant blue wrapping all around the body. This layer is the most dense, but also contains the closest connection to our Soul energy.

Second: The Emotional Layer

Location: Two to four inches away from the physical body
Correlations: Emotional energy and how we (lower personality self) feel about everything that we're experiencing in the world
Chakra: Sacral

This layer is many colors that are consistently changing according to our feelings. For example, someone who is excessively angry or lustful may have a disproportionate amount of red in this layer of their auric field, while a healthy, balanced field will look like gentle clouds ranging in the colors of the rainbow.

Third: The Mental Layer

Location: Two to four inches outside of the second layer
Correlations: How we think about everything happening in our physical reality
Chakra: Solar plexus

This layer is a beautiful bright yellow when it is clear and not clouded with excessive thoughts.

Fourth: The Astral Layer

Location: Bridge between the physical and nonphysical realms
Correlations: The energy of love
Chakra: Heart

This layer is our connection to the astral planes and is the layer of our energy that spiritually travels when we're sleeping. When healthy, it is a beautiful collection of vibrant neon pastel colors.

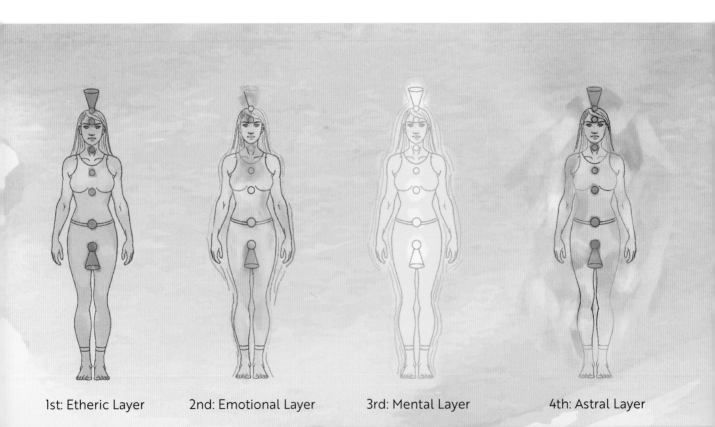

1st: Etheric Layer   2nd: Emotional Layer   3rd: Mental Layer   4th: Astral Layer

Fifth: The Etheric Template

Location: Resides in the fifth dimension
Correlations: The health and design of our physical tissues
Chakra: Throat

The etheric template is like our etheric blueprint, which is the spiritual energetic blueprint for our physical body. It literally looks like a blueprint with the similar blue energy of the first layer, but with a matrix of graph-like white lines of light intersecting through it.

When someone has surgery or a physical injury, usually this area of the aura becomes damaged. It can be tremendously helpful to speed up the patient's recovery from injury by repairing the energy in this layer of whatever organ or tissue was damaged. However, to work in these higher dimensional layers of the aura, you need to shift *your* dimensional frequency to match the layer of the aura you want to work in. So, to see and repair the fifth layer, this means you must be able to consistently, stably maintain a fifth dimensional frequency to work in and assist others in this capacity, and so forth when moving upward in the aura. This is where consistent meditation and living from the energy of love and unity comes in and becomes crucial.

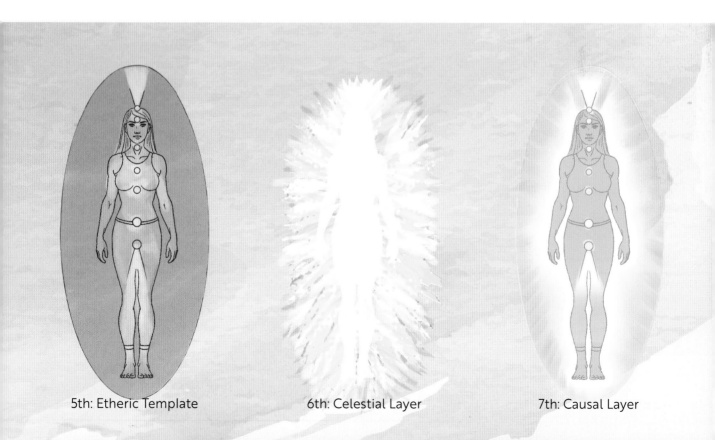

5th: Etheric Template   6th: Celestial Layer   7th: Causal Layer

Sixth: The Celestial Layer

Location: Sixth dimension
Correlations: The way our *spirit feels* about what's happening emotionally
Chakra: Third eye

Our conscious mind may feel one way about a situation, but our spirit may feel the exact opposite because it is seeing things through the eyes of compassion, from a higher dimensional perspective. The celestial layer is difficult to discern unless we are actively in touch and in communication with our spirit and understand what is occurring in this dimension. This layer is a beautiful array of gentle pastel colors.

Seventh: The Causal (Ketheric) Layer

Location: Seventh dimension
Correlations: Our spirit's thoughts and contemplations about what it's experiencing
Chakra: Crown

The seventh layer is our spirit's mental realm. This is the outermost layer (encompassing all other layers) that most energy workers and clairvoyants work with and perceive as a pure golden grid of energy. It holds the purest connection to Source energy and serves as a beautiful form of high-vibration protection when it is full of its own spiritual light.

The Vertical Power Current

Tying it all together, running down the center line of the body, just slightly in front of the spinal column, is our vertical power current, or ascension column of light. This is the center of our "tube torus field," which surrounds us at all times.

A constant exchange of information moves up and down this column, as the seven main chakras meet it at different points. The root chakra is at the very end or base of this column, the five middle chakras (correlating with each endocrine gland in the physical body) run up along this column, and the crown chakra is the funnel or vortex at the top of the column. In ancient yogic practices, the vertical power current was called the sushumna nadi in Sanskrit, or "central column," in which the kundalini energy rises up through, starting from the base of the spine, through each mastered chakra center, until it reaches the crown chakra and then enlightenment (or divine union) is attained.

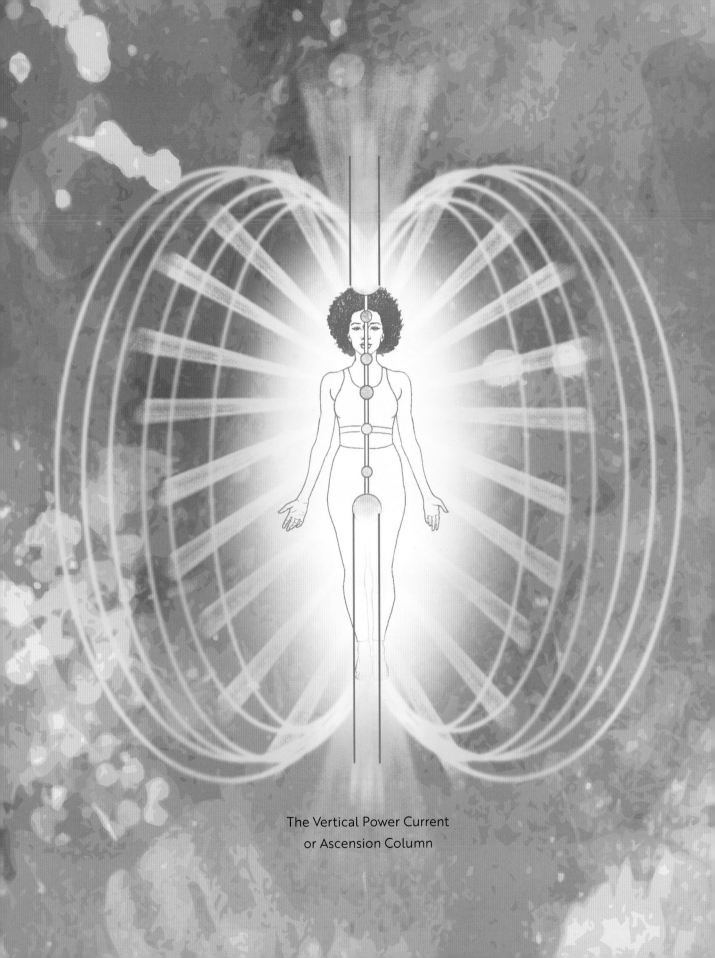

The Vertical Power Current
or Ascension Column

3

Tools to Support Your Journey

Throughout your healing journey, you can use tools and techniques to support you in your growth. They are not essential to the practice of energy healing, but they will enhance and sharpen your ability to become as clear as you can in body, mind, and spirit before beginning your practice. Use these as temporary "training wheels" to assist you, but be mindful of not relying on any one tool to the point where it becomes a crutch.

Working with Crystals

Crystals are one of my favorite energetic tools. Crystals store memory, and like a computer chip, they can be programmed to assist your spiritual experiences. In certain cases, they can recall and transmit stored information, and can even act as teachers. Think of crystals as amplification tools with their own intelligence. They are their own living, conscious beings and can be great companions on your journey to healing.

Here are just a few of the other ways crystals can help you in your practice and healing:

- Move the energy in the body quickly
- Amplify the energy where needed
- Bring in different energies for balance
- Help clear and ground your energy

Choosing the crystals you want to work with from the hundreds of forms available can be intimidating. Use one of your most important tools: your intuition. What crystal is jumping out to you visually or gives you a strong buzzing connection when you hold it? This is the one to use first.

I recommend using this intuitive technique every time you choose a new crystal for your collection: test to feel the energy of the crystal and hold it in your left hand (your receiving hand) to receive the information from it. See if you have a strong connection or not. Sometimes crystals will catch our eye or come to us, but it can take a few months or even years before we are ready to work with their energy. Often the crystals we get as gifts are the Universe's way of bringing us the ones we need most.

To use crystals for meditation, hold the crystal in your left hand or in both hands. Bring your awareness into your heart chakra through breathing, and then set the intention to connect with the crystal from the energy of your heart. As you energetically connect with the crystal, you'll activate its energy within your field. From there, release the intent and just observe: see what you receive and how you feel.

Different crystals have different purposes. If you have a hard time settling the mind, try working with a grounding crystal around your root and/or feet. Usually black, smoky, brown, or dark red crystals can assist with this. If you ground easily but feel spiritually blocked, work with the clear crystals such as quartz, or white or violet purple crystals, around your crown chakra. If you feel imbalanced in both capacities, use multiple crystals at once. You can also add in any crystal that is speaking to you by placing it in your left hand while meditating, with the intention that it works with the particular chakra or area of your energy you want to focus on.

Meditating with crystals can speed the results of your energy work. What may take an hour in meditation to release and clear can be done in fifteen to twenty minutes with your crystals. Using crystals strategically can assist with clearing or boosting your energy during your session, speeding the process, and amplifying the results. They are a powerful conduit for bringing in higher frequencies or specific energies conducive to your healing in that moment. And they're beautiful to have around your house.

Clearing and Programming Your Crystals

Unless it came straight from the ground and into your hands, a crystal needs to be cleared the first time you use it. Clearing removes the energies and programs it may have received from previous owners. There are several ways to do this, but my favorite way is to use breathing with intention.

Hold the crystal in your right hand (your giving hand). With a strong forced exhale, energetically directing your breath into the crystal, to clear the previous programs of the crystal.

If there has been serious misuse or energy collected in the crystal, you may need to take extra steps to clear it. Here are some additional techniques:

- Run the crystal under cold water while focusing on your intention to clear it. Natural water and ocean water are good options, just be careful, as sea salt can damage some crystals.
- Leave your crystal in a bowl of salt for twenty-four hours.
- Plant your crystal in the ground for twenty-four hours for the Earth to recharge and reset the energy.

Do what intuitively feels the best to you, and know that it may be different for each crystal energy that you work with.

Once your crystal is clear, it's time to program or "activate" your crystal with your intentions. The secret is first moving your awareness into your heart space. This will amplify and clearly direct the intentions, because they will be sent with the strong energy of love.

This is a simple way to program your crystals: Drop your awareness into your heart space. Hold your crystal in your right hand and set your intentions for the purpose of the crystal. Take a full powerful exhale into the crystal with the intention of programming it with these new instructions. (We will discuss a more in-depth method for programming crystals on page 123.)

When your crystal has been cleared, you can connect in to your heart again, but this time place your crystal in your left palm. Meditate and "listen" for any messages coming through from the crystal itself on how it would like to work with you.

Some crystals like to do their own thing, and others are adaptable and easily programmable. Clear quartz crystal is the easiest and highest vibration crystal to work with and program for healing. These crystals are called the "master healers" and are like the chameleons of the crystal group, as they can amplify the energy of anything you choose, including other crystals around them. Quartz are also amazing crystals for storing information and transmitting out healing energy. They can laser focus your energy when needed, and amplify the frequencies coming through them.

Crystals and the Chakras

Each chakra has different crystals that correlate with its energy. When a chakra is out of balance, it can be helpful to use crystals of that similar energy frequency to restore balance. Most crystals coordinate with chakras based on similar color energy of the chakra. There are many exceptions to this rule, as some crystals work with all of the chakras and some that do not match in color, but their energies are complementary.

Root Chakra

- Deep red or dark crystals
- Smoky quartz assists with grounding and absorbing negative energies.

Sacral Chakra

- Orange crystals
- Carnelian brings in the energy of health and vitality for the body.

Solar Plexus

- Yellow crystals
- Citrine carries the energy of joy, abundance, and confidence.

Heart Chakra

- Green or pink crystals, or crystals with a combination of the two colors
- Rose quartz brings in the gentle energy of love, and emerald brings in the energy of healing.

Throat Chakra

- Lighter and turquoise shades of blue crystals
- Aquamarine gently works on assisting us with clear communication and holds the energy of truth.

Third Eye Chakra

- Deeper blue and indigo crystals; clear crystals, such as apophyllite or diamond
- Tanzanite is a high-vibrational amplifier that assists with psychic vision and developing our intuition.

Crown Chakra

- Violet, lilac, or deep purple crystals; clear quartz and clear crystals
- Amethyst offers psychic protection and clears the mind for meditation.

More Crystals and Their Meanings

Clear quartz is a "master healer," amplifier, and generator that works with all the chakras.

Selenite is like liquid white light. It's a gentle but powerful cleanser and activator of energy. It does not need to be cleared.

Black tourmaline is similar to smoky quartz, but much stronger in frequency. It's a highly protective stone, wonderful for grounding off lower vibrations.

Blue kyanite has high-vibrational energy. It clears and rebalances all of the chakras at once. It can aid the throat and third eye chakras, and does not need to be cleared.

For powerful healing and realignment of your chakra system, simply lie down with each corresponding crystal aligned with each chakra. Or, if you have a massage table, you can lay the crystals underneath the table in alignment with your body's chakras. If you know only certain chakras need assistance, you can choose the ones that stand out the most for those areas. You can hold the crystals in your hands or by your foot chakras to bring in the healing energetic properties. You can also create a healing crystal grid or a circle around you when you lie down and meditate.

Remember to bring your awareness into your heart and concentrate on your breathing while working with crystals. When working with your crystals, it's always best to choose the method that intuitively resonates with you. And know that it's common for the crystals that resonate with you to change over time, depending on your needs and new energetic states.

Working with Sound

Harmonic sound vibration can create powerful shifts in the energetic field. Sound waves can move energy around inside the body and automatically go where they are most needed. When working with sound, you can use beautiful crystal singing bowls tuned to a particular frequency to match the chakra of your choice. You can also use one of the best, easiest, and most powerful tools available to you—your own voice.

There are tremendous spiritual benefits to adding sound vibration to your healing practice. By toning with intention, you can use the sound of your voice to send and amplify healing energy in the body quickly and easily. Ancient Sanskrit mantras like "Om," or the "Bija Mantra," moving through the chakras, can assist with clearing and balancing the energy field. Sound can also be used to clear the energy of a space, through practices like clapping or using bells or tingshas. The repetition of mantras playing in your home can also assist with lifting the vibration of your space. Playing crystal bowls can allow higher frequency beings such as angelics and spirit guides to come into your field and work with you more easily.

Music can also help if you have trouble meditating and maintaining a calm, still place of peace (which is the foundation for all successful energy healing work). Binaural beats work by creating frequencies in the brain through a process called entrainment. Working with binaural beats that can move you into alpha and then theta wave brain states are the most conducive to healing. Solfeggio frequencies were modeled after Gregorian chants, where each high-vibrational frequency has a particular effect on the energy according to its hertz vibration or cycles per second. I find these soothing to the energy field and helpful during sessions to ease into a higher vibrational, peaceful state of being. Experiment with both to see what resonates best with your practice.gifts are the Universe's way of bringing us the ones we need most.

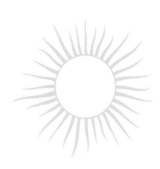

Cymatics

In physics, there is a branch of study called cymatics, where introducing sound waves onto a metal plate covered with sand naturally creates beautiful, symmetrical geometric patterns that shift according to each tone introduced. This has also been studied and shown with water. It is incredible and enlightening to see.

Our human bodies are composed of more than 60 percent water. Just as sound vibration affects sand or water to create harmonic geometric patterns out of chaotic, formless shapes, it does the same for our own energy field and waters inside, easily creating harmony in areas of disharmony.

Working with Light

The energy of photonic light can heal and replenish the energy and body. Two of the easiest, simplest ways are working with the energy of the sun and color therapy.

The sun, on a physiological level, provides so much nourishment, warmth, and energy to life on Earth. Without it, we simply wouldn't exist as a planet. On an energetic level, it sends us pure photonic light that boosts our energy field. When we spend time in the sun, vital spiritual codes come through the light. Even just ten minutes a day can have an unbelievable effect on the health and vibrancy of your aura, and on your extrasensory abilities and ability to connect with the Divine.

For centuries people have used the practice of sun gazing to connect with and take in energy from the sun into the third eye and crown chakras and their correlating glands. This is not for everyone and is typically only recommended to practice at sunrise or sunset, when the sun is at its lowest intensity, or with sunglasses on. Use your own discretion if you have sensitive eyes or just don't resonate with the practice.

Color therapy can boost your mood and energy. To begin, use your intuition and pick the colors that attract you most in the moment or in this time of your life. We usually gravitate naturally toward the colors we may be energetically depleted in—or in the case of excess, the colors that will balance or cancel out the excess opposite energy in the system. Color therapy can be explored in dozens of different ways:

- Eat particular colored foods to boost a specific chakra
- Wear a certain color clothing or jewelry
- Energetically bring that color into your energy field
- Take color baths
- Wear colored glasses
- Use specific colored crystals to bring in that color energy

In the upcoming exercises (page 106), we will go into depth on how to use color as an energetic tool in your meditation and healing sessions.

Working with Nature

As humans, we were meant to be intrinsically living in harmony with nature and her natural cycles. Our bodies actually thrive on the harmonic frequencies emitted from nature, physically and energetically. Just being in nature for twenty minutes has tremendous harmonious effects on the energy system. It is rejuvenating and grounding, and it allows our energy system and mind to slow down to a gentler frequency, similar to the resonating frequency of the Earth, the Schumann resonance, at around 7.83 hertz.

Walking barefoot or connecting your energy with the trees can be therapeutically grounding. You can also connect with nature through bringing elements of the Earth into your home. Crystals and houseplants are two easy ways to connect with the energy of nature, even if you live in an urban setting. Working with gem or flower essences is another beautiful way to bring the energy of nature into your home. See page 100 to learn more about how to energetically ground and connect with the consciousness of Gaia herself.

Working with Water

As you begin your healing practice, be conscious and mindful of everything you consume, energetically and physically. One of the easiest ways to assist energetically healing your body is through its most common element, water. You can program and structure your water (similar to the way you program crystals, see page 53). This will help amplify the water's healing benefits as it works with your body. Dr. Masaru Emoto has done a lot of research on the effect of prayer, words, and other sounds on water. Music, vibration, and energy can also affect the crystalline structure of the water.

Salt can clear and neutralize energy, and, like a magnet, it absorbs the negative energies it encounters. Here are ways to work with the healing properties of salt water:

- Swim in the ocean or take sea salt baths to clear your energetic field. Try this after a long day or after taking on or absorbing other peoples' energies or emotions.

- Make a sea salt paste with water and salt and (gently) rub it on the body over the chakra or on any area where you feel stagnation. Leave the paste on the area for a few minutes, breathing into that spot, and when you're ready, rinse it off.

- Make your own sea salt aura spray by adding sea salt to a spray bottle along with any essential oils you'd like to include. Mist it in your aura around your body wherever you'd like to clear.

Structuring and Blessing Your Water

Once you learn how to send healing energy through your hands, you'll be ready to charge and bless your water in the same way. Until that time, simply structure your water through the power of prayer. This is the same process used to create holy water. We are all divine beings and with pure heart-filled intention, we can bring the same healing energy into our water and into our lives as any other being. We don't need a middleman, as we can do this ourselves with amazing results!

Bringing your awareness into your heart, hold the water glass in your hands or place your hands above the water.

Set the intention that this water is now energetically purified and divinitized. Charge it with the energy of pure divine love or peace, or any high-vibrational energy you'd like.

Thank the water for its healing properties, and then simply take a breath. Open your eyes and take a sip!

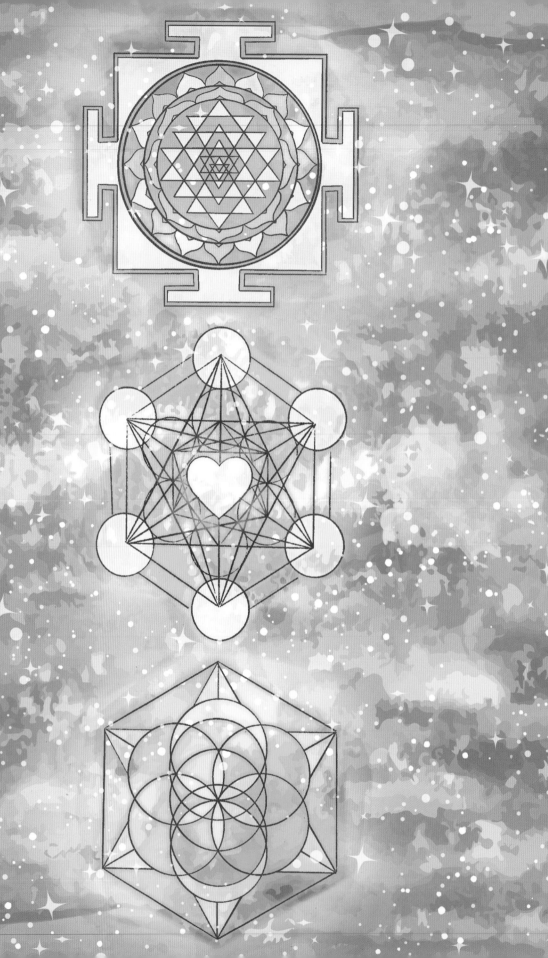

Working with Sacred Geometry and Sacred Symbols for Healing

Working with sacred geometry is a science and an art form. By briefly working with, meditating on, or looking at drawings of sacred geometric symbols, we can help reawaken memories of our cosmic and ancient origins as energy before entering the physical body. Beautiful symbols are wonderful places to start: try the seed of life, the flower of life, Metatron's cube, the Merkabah, and the Sri Yantra (considered the most powerful symbol). Gaze at the images on this page and just let your eyes follow the connecting lines and patterns. When our clairvoyance activates, many of us will see these repeating sacred geometric patterns in our inner vision as they are activating those gifts.

Another favorite ancient symbol is the Antahkarana, which is a bridge or connector to the energy of your higher self. Meditate with the symbol under your seat or feet. It can create the connection, bring more energy from your higher self down into the body, and boost healing.

The Benefit of Movement and Exercise for Your Energy

Exercise is *as important* for your energy as it is for your physical health. Daily movement will circulate the energy in the body in the same way that it circulates blood flow. With simple exercise and mindful movement practices, such as walking, yoga, tai chi, and dance, you can speed up and improve your energy healing results. Healthy exercise can help move and ground off energies that are no longer serving you. The key to amplifying the healing effect of the movement practice is to always set the intention and then move with conscious awareness, as if you were in a moving prayer or meditation during your exercise.

These tools assist you with your healing practice along the way. You can use all or a few, but these tools are amazing ways to assist and boost your already naturally gifted skills. Turning these practices into routines can be a beautiful way to show self-love and assist in your healing journey. These are all ideally meant to be used as tools, meaning items that can help or support your journey, but not as crutches, where you become dependent on one or more of these items to do your spiritual work. Ideally, all we need is our breathing and our body to create the most healing energetic sessions for ourselves in the long run.

PART

II

THE
PREPARATION

In this section, we dive into the profound practices of conscious breathwork and meditation to get familiar with our own true energy within. You'll work through simple exercises that will move you into parasympathetic mode to prepare your energy for the deeper exercises. You can incorporate these exercises into your daily routine for the overall wellness of your mind, body, and spirit. Then, we'll talk about how to clear your space, find a ritual to get yourself and your space ready, and set your intentions before you begin an energy healing session.

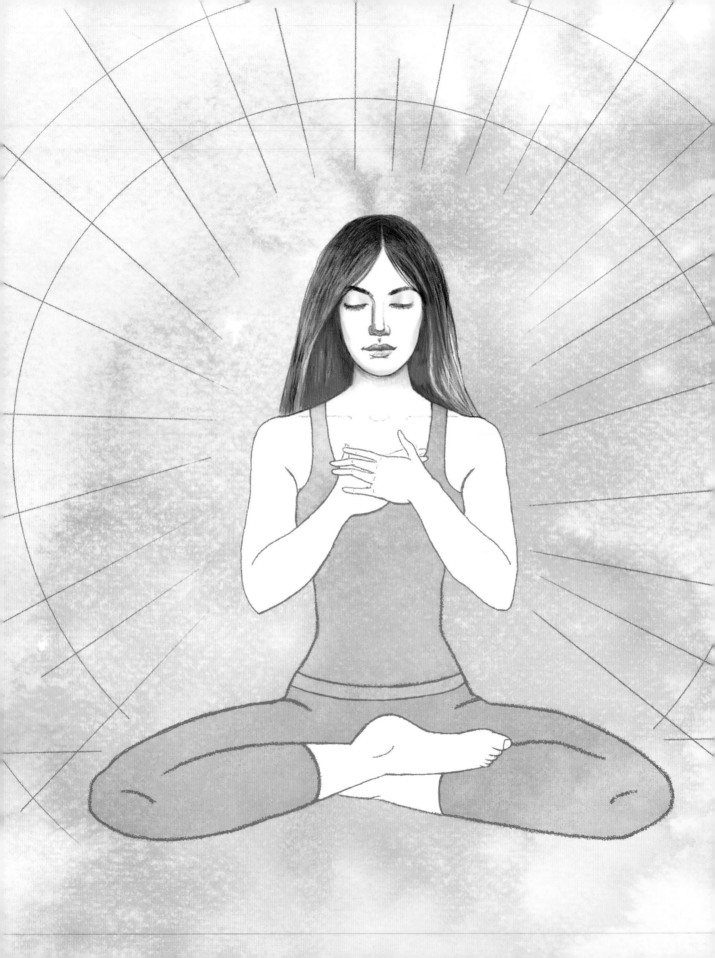

4

Exercises to Prepare Your Energy

This chapter is all about preparing the energy. The exercises help us get to know our own energy and internal resources, working from the inside out. All you'll need is a comfortable place to sit, a journal, your body, and your breath—that's it!

We'll begin by learning simple, easy breath exercises and meditation techniques that will support your practice. An energy session for thirty minutes to an hour means you will keep the energy flowing continuously in that time. The best way to prepare to do this without getting distracted is daily meditation. This will assist your energy healing practice in so many ways, and allow you to dive deeper into sessions with more clarity and focus.

Retraining Your Nervous System

A huge part of energy healing is working with your breath to move the energy through your system. Your breath, along with your intention, can consciously guide and alter the flow of energy throughout the channels in your system.

When working with energy, make sure that you are in a calm and relaxed place before the start of each session. The energetic state you're in can steer the direction of your work and assist or hinder the results. It is especially important when moving, amplifying, and bringing in energy that you are in a calm, neutral place and not angry or fearful. Bringing yourself to a calm, neutral place involves actively retraining your nervous system. You do not need to be a longtime yogi or Zen master to work with energy, but you should be able to keep your cool for a few hours throughout the day.

The two main aspects of the nervous system that you'll need to know are the sympathetic nervous system (or "fight or flight" mode) and the parasympathetic nervous system (or "rest and digest" mode). These systems operate under the autonomic branch of the nervous system, which operates unconsciously to regulate bodily functions such as our heart rate, breathing, and digestion. It keeps working while we're not thinking about it, and also controls whether we are in a high-alert, anxious state or in relaxed, calm state.

The sympathetic nervous system (SNS) is activated during stressful events or moments requiring you to be on high alert. It's also triggered by stimulants, such as having too much coffee. There is an increase in the heart rate, blood pressure, and adrenaline; most of the blood is moved out into the extremities, diverted away from the gut and reasoning centers of the brain.

The parasympathetic nervous system (PNS) is switched on when there is no longer any sign of perceived danger and we feel like we're safe so we can relax again. Our heart rate slows down and our blood pressure is lowered. The secretion of adrenaline is turned off. Digestion is turned on because the blood flow is now being sent to the gut and the reasoning centers of the brain. Some signs the PNS is active are yawning, taking deep, sigh exhales, swallowing, tummy gurgles, and deep relaxation.

Typically, we have no conscious awareness or control over the functions of our autonomic nervous system. In a healthy nervous system, we are primarily in the PNS throughout the day. Here and there, we move quickly into SNS mode, and then quickly back out of it. However, when we are faced with everyday stressors that never seem to turn off or disappear, this ends up reversed.

We can work with this unconscious system to regulate how we feel and which state we reside in. Learning how to train and soothe your nervous system can be an invaluable tool for regulating your energy. Two of the best ways to start are working with your breath and beginning a short meditation practice. Both are free, easy to learn, and highly effective.

Alternative ways to move into "rest and digest" mode:

- Take a yoga class
- Get acupuncture
- Spend time in nature
- Spending time off relaxing
- Breathwork and meditation

With our conscious awareness and effort, we can move the body into PNS mode in as quickly as a few short minutes.

When we consciously relax, our energetic channels naturally open, so our energy can flow freely and healthily throughout the body. Just through the simple act of relaxation, we give our energy—and thus our body—the chance to naturally heal itself.

As you'll learn in the coming chapters and exercises, relaxing prepares the body for energy healing and it *starts the process*. Energy blocks, cords, and thoughtforms hanging around in the aura can even be dissolved and released through a simple relaxation practice without any conscious effort.

Exercise: Diaphragmatic Breathing

Diaphragmatic breathing, or deep belly breathing, is one of the simplest ways to deepen your breathing, increase your oxygen levels, and regulate the nervous system. It stimulates the vagus nerve and lowers your anxiety.

The diaphragm is a dome-shaped muscle that sits below the lungs. When we breathe in, our belly expands and the diaphragm expands downward, widens, and flattens out. When we breathe out, our belly naturally draws in. The diaphragm domes back up into its jelly-fish-looking resting shape.

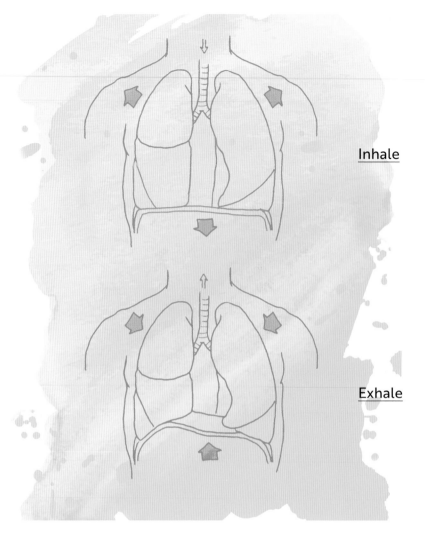

Inhale

Exhale

Diaphragmatic Breathing

This movement of the diaphragm occurs naturally and properly when the belly is moving along with the breathing (see page 70). If the abdomen is tight or contracted and we're only using our ribs, upper chest, and collarbones to breathe, then the diaphragm is not given the space it needs to move naturally. This inhibiting of true "deep breathing" limits the amount of oxygen being brought into the body, which commonly triggers the SNS. When moving into a calm, relaxed state, it's important to practice slow and deep diaphragmatic breathing. Let's learn how.

Take a few normal breaths and notice how your body is moving. Observe how you feel in this moment.

When ready, lie down on the floor, flat on your back. Bend your knees so you can plant your feet flat on the floor. Separate your feet about two feet apart, and let the knees fall together so they touch. This position with the legs—also called half-savasana—allows space for more neutral curves in the spine.

Place your hands on your belly, right around the navel.

Breathing through the nose for the entire exercise, take a slow, deep breath into the location of your hands. Feel your belly expand as the hands widen (your diaphragm is descending and widening). Slowly exhale, letting the belly draw back in as the hands come closer together (your diaphragm is doming back up to neutral). Note that the upper chest and collarbones aren't actively involved in this breathing.

Now add a little pressure with your hands onto the belly. Put gentle pressure on the belly and slowly breathe into your hands, using your abdomen to push the hands wider apart. Then slowly breathing out, use slight pressure to draw the belly back in. Repeat this a few times, until you no longer need the pressure of your hands assisting you and your belly naturally expands as you inhale and draws in as you exhale.

Once you're ready, come back up to a comfortable sitting position. Make sure your back is supported by a pillow or chair. This helps maintain its natural curves again so you don't need to engage any supporting muscles to sit upright.

Try this same belly breathing exercise, using slight pressure with your hands. After a few rounds, release the pressure, and when ready, release the hands too—but maintain the deep, diaphragmatic belly breathing for at least a minute, or as long as you can.

Now return to your normal breathing. Notice what your breath is like in this moment and how you feel after a few, simple rounds of diaphragmatic breathing.

Although this seems simple—and it is—breathing in this new way can be challenging for people if they have held a different breathing pattern their whole life. Working with belly breathing can retrain twenty, thirty, or even forty years of unconscious shallow breathing.

If this was a challenging exercise, take your time to practice it daily and especially in times of stress. Try setting an alarm on your phone to remind you to check in with your breathing, even if it's for two minutes at a time. If after a few weeks it's still challenging, I would recommend taking up a yoga practice that involves stretching the torso or seeking a breathwork specialist or physical therapist who can work on releasing tension in the diaphragm.

Adopt this simple breathing practice for one to three minutes any time you'd like to move from a sympathetic state into a relaxed and calm parasympathetic state.

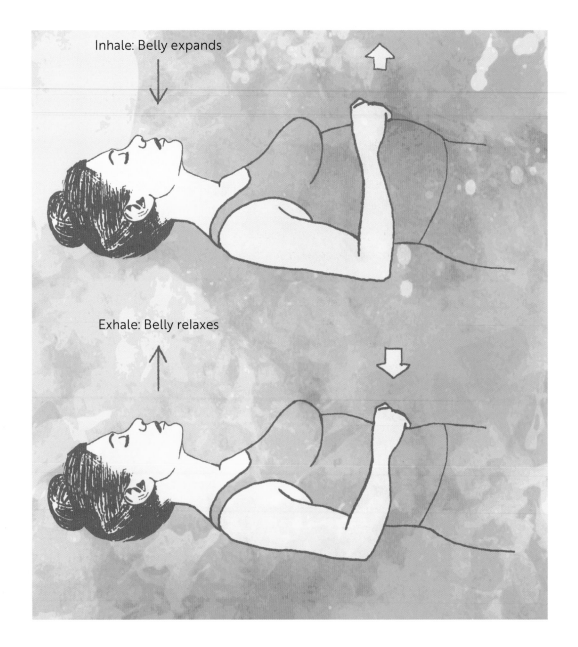

Inhale: Belly expands

Exhale: Belly relaxes

Exercise: Mind-Centering Concentration

Building on the last exercise, we will add counting the breath to even out its rhythm. This practice centers the mind and moves us deeper into a state of relaxation. The length of our inhale and exhale matters: when we're stressed, we take larger inhales and shorter exhales. When we're tired or relaxed, we do the opposite. The key is to even out the length of our inhale to the length of our exhale. This exercise is a yogic pranayama (the Sanskrit word for breath control) technique called *sama vritti*, or equal part breathing.

Find a comfortable seat where your spine is supported and in its natural curves.

Take three slow, diaphragmatic breaths, in and out.

Add slow counts to your next inhale. Inhale for 4 seconds, counting mentally: 1...2...3...4.

Then exhale for 4 seconds, counting mentally: 1...2...3...4. (That's one round.)

Repeat this breathing with even counting for the next two minutes (about twelve more rounds). Remember to breathe diaphragmatically as you're counting, and once you get the hang of it close your eyes.

When you finish, open your eyes and notice how you feel.

This exercise regulates the nervous system and works on concentrating the mind, which helps us take a break from the never-ending thought stream.

––––––––

If you enjoyed this exercise, aim to practice sama vritti for about five minutes every day, and if you didn't enjoy it, make it ten. (Just kidding.) It's an amazing preparation for the body and the mind before moving onto our next step, mindful meditation.

Exercise: Guided Mindful Meditation

If you're at a level where you can reach stillness and relaxation fairly easily, you can do this meditation exercise on its own. If you're just starting out and you've practiced the previous exercises consecutively, you're most likely already in a decently relaxed state. That is *perfect* for energy healing. Now let's continue until you hit the "sweet spot," where you're peaceful and it feels like time doesn't matter or exist. (Yes, this *is* very possible to achieve regularly through a daily meditation practice—but it *does* take time and consistency.)

To get the most out of this meditation, prerecord it on your phone or device and play it back so you can keep your eyes closed the whole time. Or you can follow along by taking a peek at each line. Either way is great. This meditation should take five to ten minutes. Let's begin.

Find a comfortable seat with your feet flat on the floor. Take three deep, diaphragmatic breaths. When you're ready, close your eyes.

Bring your awareness to the sounds around you, near and far. Notice the drones, the hums, and the intermittent sounds of your external reality. Take a few moments here.

Now bring your awareness into the body, as we do a light, three-dimensional scan. Scan down your body, starting at the top of the head, becoming fully aware of how you're feeling physically in this moment, without judgment.

Move down past the forehead, jaw, and neck. If you notice any tension, simply acknowledge it, or relax it, and then keep moving on. Scan down the shoulders and the arms, into the hands on your lap.

Scan down your torso, abdomen, and pelvis. Scan down past your seat, into your legs, moving past the knees, ankles, and into the feet. Become very aware of the connection of your feet on the floor.

Open up the chakras on the soles of your feet through your simple intention or visualization. Visualize growing energetic "roots" down below you into the Earth. Allow these roots to grow as wide as they are deep, and just breathe here for a few moments.

Bring your awareness to your breathing and gently move into mentally counting the breath (sama vritti) for a minute or two, to regulate your inhales and exhales.

Let go of the counting, and simply remain aware of your breathing. Notice the rise and fall of your breath, notice the sound and gentle movement of your body. Just *be here* for a minute or two.

When ready, take a deep breath and bring your awareness back into your body. Take a moment here.

Gently shift your awareness back onto the sounds around you, noticing them all around.

When you're ready, gently open your eyes. Take a moment just to pause here and notice how you're feeling in this moment.

When you're ready, log and journal your experience.

This simple meditation exercise can train your mind and conscious awareness into the fullness of the present moment. It's a powerful tool to silence the thoughts and bring you into a calmer and more peaceful place.

This meditation style is more mentally active than some others, but it's an amazing way to train the mind. Practice this meditation daily for a few days before moving to the next exercise. This will help move you into the parasympathetic system and train the mind, so you'll be able to maintain longer periods of mental focus and clarity with your meditation practice.

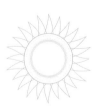

Exercise: Sitting in the Silence

You have worked with the body, breath, and mind. Now you will work with the spirit, or your energy or essence, through silence. Sitting in silence sounds like the simplest exercise of them all, but it can actually be the most challenging and most advanced form of meditation there is, especially when practiced for extended periods of time.

In the stillness of silence we can discover what lies beneath the surface, and discover and know our true inner energy. This is also where the untamed and unaddressed thoughts may rise to the surface, and you may be surprised by what you find. These thoughts typically arise to be acknowledged consciously, so they can then be released from your energy field. In this sense, sitting in silence is similar to emptying the bin, clearing the search history, or even brushing your teeth every day. The more clearing you do *now*, and the more consistently you meditate, the less you'll have to deal with later while working energetically. This will make your energy healing practice run much more efficiently.

When we meditate in silence and get the body into this relaxed and peaceful state, we are naturally bringing so much light into our energy fields. We connect with our energy, our spirit, and universal oneness, or power, and this helps boost our overall light quotient and energy. It is very similar to plugging in your phone to charge it—your energy will be cleaner and brighter, making your work ten times easier.

If you are brand new to meditation and the last exercise was your first taste of it, then continue to practice the last exercise, and each time begin to add on periods of time in silence after you've been following the breath: this can be adding on two minutes of silence each day, eventually building it up to five or ten minutes. If you already have some form of a consistent meditation practice, then move on to this next exercise.

Find a comfortable seat where your spine can maintain its natural curves.

Set a timer on your phone, clock, or app for five minutes. Before starting it, take a few slow, deep diaphragmatic breaths. If the mind is more active today, then take a few moments to practice the equal-part breathing with counting (see page 71).

When you're ready, let the counting and concentrated breathing practice go, and start your timer.

Close your eyes and allow yourself just to sit in silence for this time, noticing and neutrally observing what comes up, but not attaching to the thoughts or reacting to them emotionally. Just allow those thoughts to come and go, like clouds passing in the sky.

Each time you follow a train of thought, bring yourself back to the breath for a moment, and then back to the silence, shifting back to the seat of an observer each time.

Once the timer goes off, take a moment to slowly open your eyes and notice how you feel.

When you're ready, log and journal your experience.

———————

Sitting in silence can bring up a lot. For some people, this may allow them to drop right into a feeling of peace. But for most, this practice is where the highest degree of mental discipline and spiritual maturity can be tested and attained. Learning to train and discipline the mind allows us to sit through all sorts of storms in our physical reality, and remain a lot more neutral and observational when things come up in our energy field during our practice. There are always exceptions, but it is very normal to spend weeks, months, or even years clearing energetic remnants through this meditation practice, before getting to the more peaceful place with ease.

This practice also allows us to connect deeply with our spirit. This is where you may feel, sense, or know the loving presence of peace within, or essentially, who you truly are inside. These moments of connection become stronger and more frequent once you give your meditation practice the conscious attention it deserves. Each time this connection is made, it strengthens your energy, boosts your auric field, and fills you up with more light. These are beautiful ways to raise your energetic frequency quickly, and will make your energy healing practice flow with more ease and grace.

Exercise: Gratitude to Raise Your Vibration

Gratitude is a simple practice that can elevate and shift your mood and energy almost instantly. It's the simple art of showing appreciation for the way things *are*. Gratitude is the heartfelt way of saying "thank you" to all that is and for all that you *already have*. It doesn't take much time to build up to or require the same discipline that a meditation practice may need, but it can create such profound energetic shifts. Gratitude also changes your overall mood and energy, which will improve your practice and accelerate your abilities as a healer. You can feel the effects instantly, and a consistent practice can be life-changing.

Take a moment to get an overall picture of your mood in this moment.

Grab your journal and create a "Gratitude Practice" entry.

Start with listing five things you are grateful for and why. It is helpful to start each sentence with "I am so grateful and thankful for . . ." For example: "I am so grateful and thankful for my houseplants because they clean the air in my home and bring me a sense of joy in my heart when I see them."

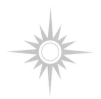

When you've completed listing your five things, list five more.

Now take a moment to just sit, place your hands over your heart, and feel the love and appreciation radiating out from your heart center.

Stay here, breathing with this feeling for as long as you can.

When you're ready, gently open your eyes, and notice your mood now. Has it shifted? Journal your experience.

––––––––––

The practice of gratitude shifts us into a higher, energetic state—one where we are so thankful for what we already have that it opens our hearts and thus opens us to receiving even more. Energetically, it acts like a magnet, attracting to us more and more of these similar high vibrations of love, thankfulness, and appreciation in our lives.

Each emotion has a resonating frequency, similar to sound waves or color frequencies; some are low and slow, and some are high and fast. You can think of your emotional energy as having its own pulse or charge to it—positive, negative, or neutral. There is no judgment as to where you are in each moment. The value is in becoming *aware* of your emotional state and how it affects your daily perceived experience.

This gratitude practice acts as a tool to help move us up the emotional ladder, from a lower or negative state into a more neutral or higher positive frequency. When practicing energy healing, we should be starting with an emotionally neutral to positive emotional state. When we amplify and move our energy around, "like attracts like," and we'll be bringing in and attracting to us experiences of similar resonating frequencies to that of our starting point. Practice this gratitude exercise daily, especially in the morning, to set the tone for your day, lift your emotional frequency, and raise your overall energetic vibration.

Take your time working with these exercises. Use them to strengthen, clarify, and purify your energy field. Get comfortable with working with your mind, body, and spirit so you feel energized and confident moving into your first self-guided energy healing session. Every individual is unique and will have different amounts of time needed for each practice and will resonate with different exercises at different points in their journey. There is no rush to the finish line (or to the next chapter). The benefit of learning and growth comes from the experience itself.

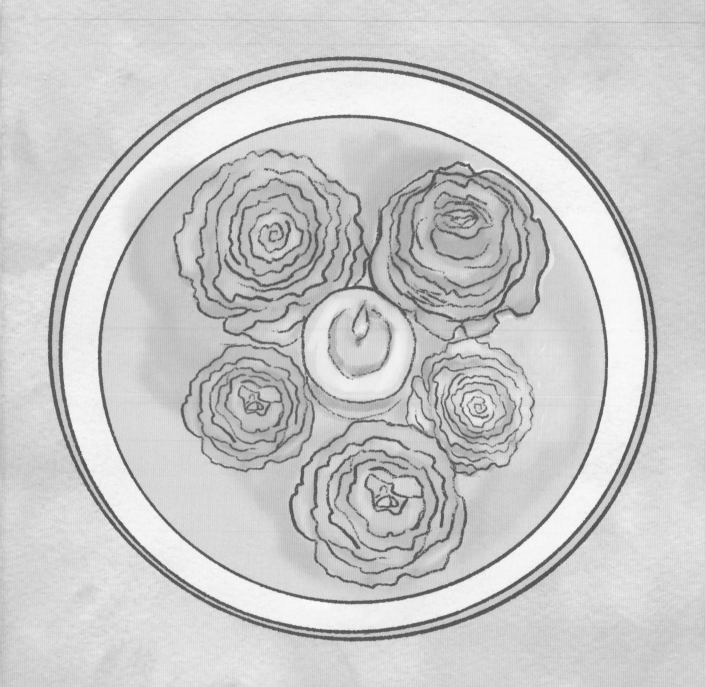

5

Setting Up for Energy Healing and Creating Sacred Space

Before working with energy healing, it is especially important to energetically clear and prepare your physical space. Our space has its own vibration, or consciousness. Just as the rooms of your home can physically collect dust bunnies in the corners, they can also collect energetic "dust" or lower, stagnant, emotional energy in spaces and in furniture. These pockets of "dirty energy" can influence the efficacy and purity of energy coming in and being moved around our own system as we overlay our aura within our environment.

Clearing Your Space

Before sitting down to work with energy or meditate, take time to clean, clear, and lift the vibration of your space. It will greatly improve your abilities and success rate when working with energy. There are simple, easy ways that we can clear the old energy in our space and make our homes a living sanctuary. On a very basic level, clutter is a magnet for accumulating negative energy in the home. So before doing the next *energetic* steps, physically clear the clutter and old piles of stuff around the home: this can be clutter in the fridge, the mail, your closet, and *especially* the space that you'll be spending most of your time in while doing deep meditation work and energy healing. The space should be clutter free and clean and clear of dust and dirt.

It is also helpful to remove any old or low-vibrational items from your healing space, as everything has an energy to it. Darker images from scary movies, images of violence, posters with curse words, and things like this can also severely lower the frequency of your space. Add uplifting images or items that bring you joy and inspiration to raise the frequency of your space. For example, add fresh flowers, houseplants, crystals, spiritual quotes, pictures of sacred geometry, archangels, ascended masters, unicorns, or high vibrational energies that you resonate with.

Simple practices to clear the *energy* of the home are passed down through ancient ceremonies, but are now common in our everyday life. Smudging or "saging" our homes with white sage, cedarwood, or palo santo is an effective, easy way to movie, clear, or sweep out old energy. White sage is the strongest form of clearing and palo santo brings positive energy into the space, but both can clear the space. It's important when saging to open the windows and allow the smoke that's accumulated the collected energy to move out—and you can do this with a fan or a feather.

An important key to making this practice effective is setting the intention to do so *beforehand*. So, you can state out loud that you are "clearing the energy of this space—all lower energies must go now."

Another option is to use sound, such as clapping, singing bowls, mantras, symbols, gongs, or tingshas. Again, it's crucial that you set the intention beforehand. Loud clapping really "breaks up" and pushes out the stagnant energy and can be a simple, powerful tool, which is why sound-based fireworks have been used in many Asian and Eastern cultures to drive away old energy and allow for the new.

Essential oils are also a beautiful way to help clear and raise the vibration of your space. You can create an essential oil spray with some sea salt mixed into it to clear the energy. Diffusing oils such as spearmint or peppermint can also help clear the energy in the space. Oils such as lavender, rose, and frankincense can tremendously lift the vibration of the space after it has been cleared, as will lighting incense or candles.

The Power of Ritual

Once you work with energy, there is a lot of power to creating and having your own personal ritual. Going through the same process signifies to the body consciousness and the mind and spirit (your personal energy and the energy around you) that you are ready to move into a higher dimensional frequency and connect inward with your own energy field.

Consider the following possibilities and then choose a ritual of your own to do before you start each healing session.

- Place rose or frankincense blended oil on your third eye, light a candle, and say a prayer to the highest power to watch over your space.

- Light incense and put on your favorite soothing playlist to move you into the healing "zone."

- Offer a flower to a meditation altar or space in your home, or set up a crystal grid around you, and take a few deep breaths before beginning.

- Use a meditation shawl around your shoulders.

Performing a sacred ritual that is personal and inspiring to you will create a patterning that signals to your energy (and your guides) that it's time to start the healing work. Experiment with different options and see what resonates most with your energy, according to what opens your heart and easily moves you into a state of peace.

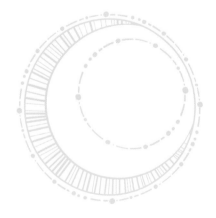

Setting Intentions

Setting your intention is a powerful way of directing the energy to flow toward a particular path. In healing sessions, it's possible that most of the healing work can be done just through the power of initially setting an intention (not always, but much of the time).

You can set new intentions each day, or stick with the same ones for a few days or weeks until they manifest in your life. Some examples of intentions are:

*I now intend to release all lower emotional energy
that I may be storing in my system.*

I now intend to release all energy that is not mine.

*I now intend to rebalance and heal my
entire chakra system.*

*I now set the intention to fill the energy of my heart with
the divine frequency of unconditional love.*

I now intend to fill every cell of my body with light.

You can set any intentions that come from your heart. Take a moment before each session to take a few deep, diaphragmatic breaths, slow down your heart rate (and thus, your mind), and bring your awareness into your heart center. Then flow with the intentions that come to you in that space. You can even set this intention before you begin: "I now only work with the intentions that lovingly move me on the path toward my highest good. And so it is."

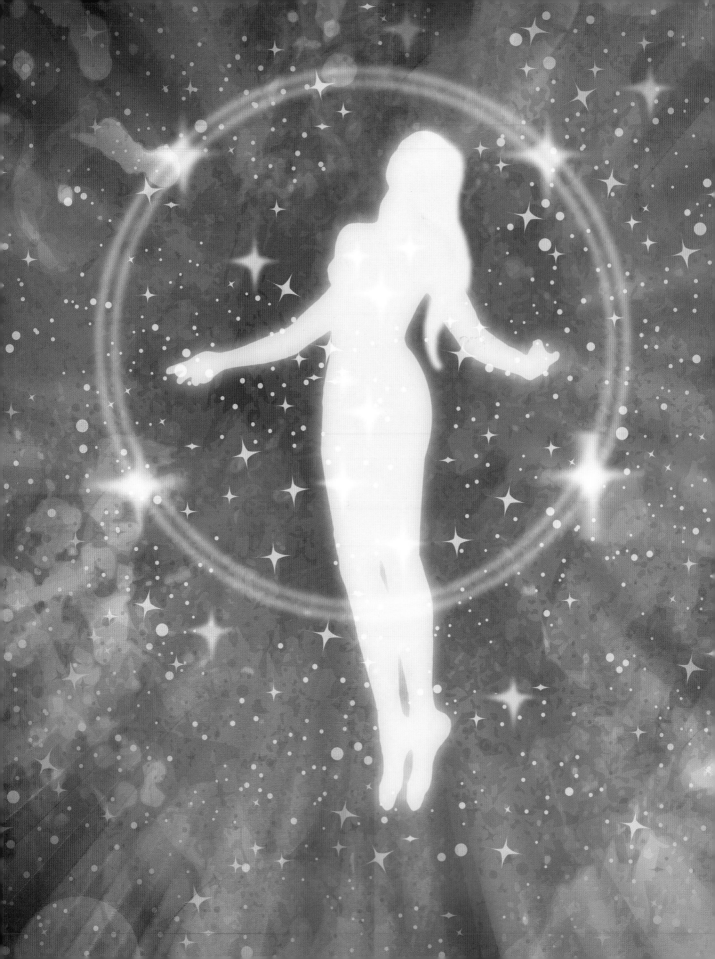

6

Things You May Experience During Energy Healing

B efore you work with energy, it's important to know there are potential energetic sensations that may occur during the process. This chapter covers some of the possibilities before diving in, so you firmly understand what's occurring. The following are common responses to energy work, but everyone experiences them differently; it all depends on the individual's sensitivity level to energy, which will develop and bloom. And while the experiences aren't limited to what's included here, there are some pretty standard responses to energy work.

Common Responses to Energy Work

Initially, as your sensitivity develops, you may feel light currents of electricity moving through the channels. This isn't painful and is usually very mild. Getting the "chills" or goosebumps during your sessions or while setting intentions is usually a beautiful thing. This is a crystallization of the etheric DNA happening when your Soul resonates with something it has heard (and has now "remembered") or when your spiritual energy begins entraining and vibrating with a higher frequency energy.

When the energy work you're doing is primarily based on charging, boosting, or filling an area, you may experience the sensation of heat or warmth around that area. When the energy work you're doing is primarily focused around clearing old or stagnant energy from your system, it's likely you'll experience a very icy or cooling sensation in all the areas being cleared.

During sessions it is also fairly common to experience emotional releases of older stored emotions rising to the surface to be flushed out, some peaceful and some less so. This can occur beautifully as crying, usually in the case of a deep healing and release. Old anger, grief, or sadness can release as well, leaving room to experience greater states of happiness, bliss, and divine peace. Usually the lower emotion stepping up is one that's been dormant or repressed and has finally been given an outlet during your healing session. Holding a space of nonjudgment and compassion for yourself during these cathartic moments is key.

It's also possible to have dreamlike visions, thoughts, pictures, colors, or symbols appear during your sessions. Some of these are the energies that are being cleared that you can now witness. Others are the energies coming in to boost your field. And after working with clearing and strengthening your energy field (until it achieves stability), some people may receive telepathic messages and experience feelings of love and support from their higher selves or team of spirit guides.

For most people, energy healing occurs during the session and leaves you in a deeply relaxed theta brain wave state. Occasionally during personal sessions or guided sessions (initially), it's common for the person to fall asleep (moving past theta and going directly into delta). This doesn't happen to everyone, but usually when it does there is deep healing in the energy field and body and the spirit itself pops up safely out of the body to witness what's occurring and assist. When this occurs, you'll feel the effects of the session afterward, but you will not retain the conscious information of what occurred during the healing. This will happen less and less the more you practice remaining consciously aware in these relaxed states during your meditation practice, as you can hold more light in the body each time. This is why a meditation practice is a key ingredient in the recipe for a successful healing practice.

Your Energetic Sensitivity Levels

Some people also may not feel anything—not a single thing—during a session. In these cases, whether they are receiving a session from a professional or doing the session themselves, *the energy healing work is still happening*. They just have not yet developed their sensitivity to the energy yet.

This can occur for many reasons:

- Poor nutrition leading to chemical imbalances
- Physical or psychological ailments, such as depression
- Prolonged use of particular prescription medications
- Regular use of narcotics or excessive use of alcohol
- Severe childhood trauma or sexual trauma
- Anything that creates excessive damage to the physical tissues or energy body at any age

This can lead to the individual's body shutting down their sensory system to numb the pain. Sensitivity can be easy to heal and develop—or it can take months of energy work.

If you find a lack of sensitivity even after following the exercises in this book for a few months, try engaging in professional energy healing services. Deeper clearing and repair may be needed, along with following a healthy and moderate detox program, while improving nutrient intake. Seek the care of your medical doctor before changing your daily diet.

Most people do develop profound sensitivity in their body and hands as the energy shifts in their system within a few sessions or weeks of using the practices we discuss here. And some may have profound experiences even during their first session. The most important thing is to leave your expectations at the door and be open to feeling, sensing, hearing, and knowing the unique shifts occurring in your present moment. Each session you do will be unique in its own right. Be open and embrace the process.

Functional Integration

At the end of each session, there is a period that Russell Forsyth from the IEL Institute for the Spiritual Arts has termed *functional integration*: the body takes a certain amount of time to adjust and recalibrate from the shift in energy. A functional integration period from a session could last a few short hours or days, weeks, months—or in some rare cases with deeper work done, years.

This is a key part of the healing process and can be just as important as the energy healing itself. It is the time you allow for your body to readjust to the new energetic alignments and new light levels that have entered the body. It can occasionally cause people to be moody and need extra rest, while also simultaneously feeling happier and "lighter" than ever. Energy healing happens in layers, so as we work with and move one layer of the energy during the integration period, previously uncovered layers can come to the surface. This is also why we can sometimes feel worse before we feel better.

During the integration period, it's also possible for the body to experience physical symptoms, such as minor aches, pains, and cold-like symptoms, because as we remove the toxic energy from our system, the toxic cells that resonated with that energy also begin to clear. Most people can feel fine, and often much better, after doing a session. Again, always check with your medical doctor if physical symptoms persist.

During each integration period, rehydrate with lots of water and electrolytes because the body becomes depleted when the energy is being moved during and after a session. It is also a beautiful time to be gentle with yourself and engage in extra self-care practices to assist the healing.

Remember to pace yourself and take each session and integration period step by step. Adding too much energy work too quickly can overload the system and hinder or shift the work that has already been done. This can also potentially lead to a healing crisis, where serious physical and psychological issues can occur if too much work is done too soon.

Slow and steady is definitely the best way to approach your healing journey. It is a *journey*, with nuggets of wisdom and understanding learned with each step taken. It is most definitely not a race to a single final destination or finish line. Keep in mind that even beyond this physical incarnation, we are eternal beings and will always be continuously growing and ascending our energies in the higher spiritual planes.

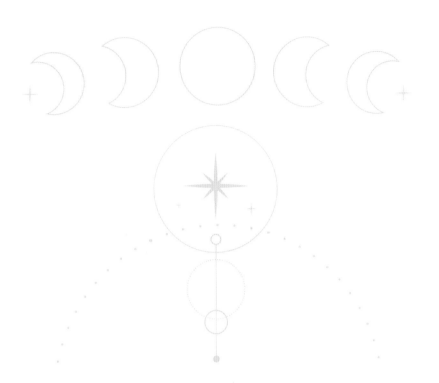

"Energy healing happens in layers, so as we work with and move one layer of the energy during the integration period, previously uncovered layers can come to the surface. This is also why we can sometimes feel worse before we feel better."

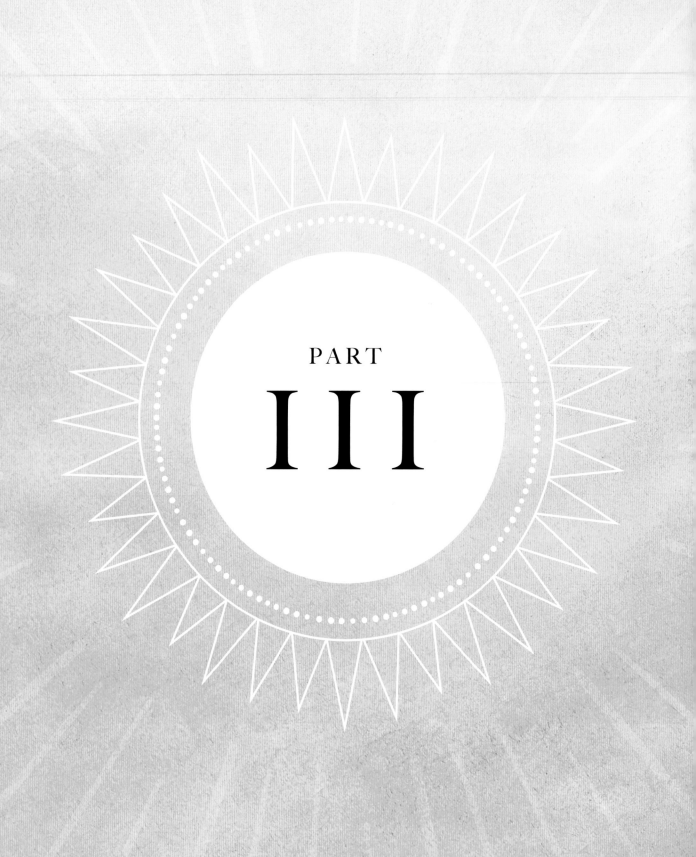

PART

III

ENERGY HEALING TECHNIQUES AND EXERCISES

As you begin practicing energy healing, you'll start to see how far you've already come. You've gained an understanding of your energy anatomy. You've been meditating daily, and you're undergoing any lifestyle shifts needed to prepare you for this very moment. Congratulations!

Working with energy is such a beautiful, sacred art form. Many people go through their entire lives without knowing its value, simply because it was not in their awareness. But you have seen beyond that veil. It is my firm belief that there are no coincidences in our universe, and the fact that you are beginning your energy healing journey in this very moment is exactly where you are supposed to be. Take your time as you work through the exercises and learn about yourself and your energy. Remember that you are a beautiful being of light, and enjoy the process!

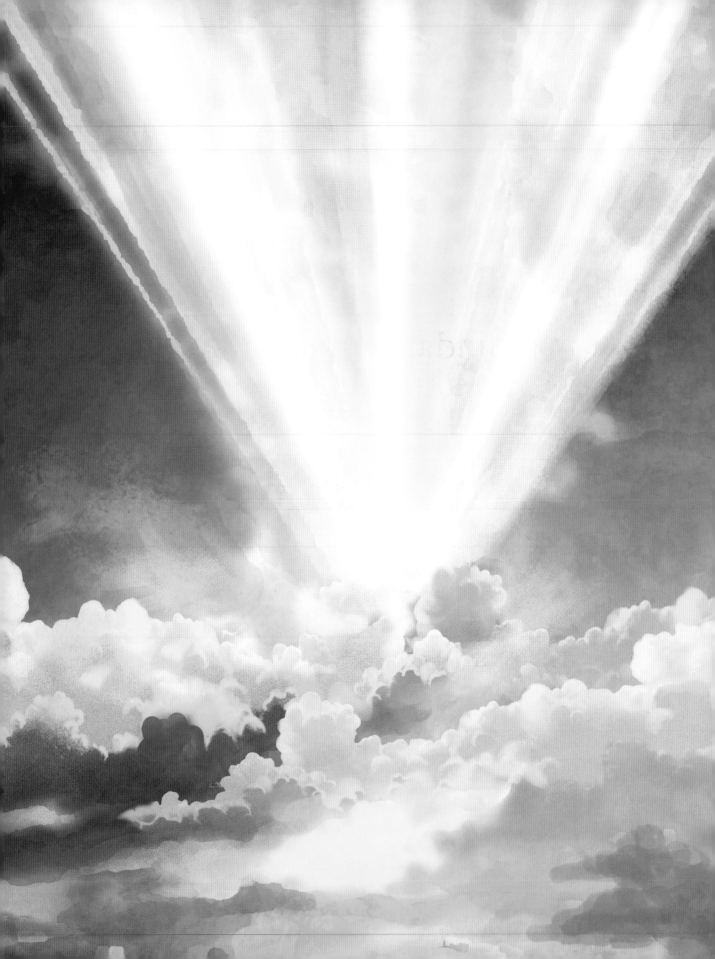

7

Foundational Energy Healing Practices

It's here! Now is the moment that you've been waiting for and working toward since starting this book. You've read all the anatomy, you've been meditating daily, you've studied for hours and hours (maybe not, but we're on a roll here), and you've undergone all of the *major* lifestyle changes and shifts needed to prepare you for this very moment. Congratulations! The preparation work to get you here was about half of the work on its own. Now it's time to get into the juicy stuff and begin *actually practicing energy healing.*

Each exercise in this foundational chapter will build upon the last. You'll know you're ready to move forward when you've had a *tangible*, distinguishable, energetic experience that you saw, felt, sensed, or heard from that exercise. Then, you'll want to become proficient in the technique by repeating the exercise and achieving the same (or similar) results again and again.

Shifting Your Energy for Healing

Working with energy is such a beautiful, sacred art form. Most people go through their entire lives not having any idea of its value or existence, simply because it was not in their awareness. But you have already seen beyond that veil, and the thing that drew you to this book is finally here. Consider this your first year at Hogwarts, and you're about to walk through platform 9¾.

Going through the exercises in this chapter can take anywhere from a few days to a few months to master. A strong foundation for your energy work is absolutely essential: *take your time with each exercise.* Each technique builds upon the last; just as when building a house, you need a strong, sturdy foundation. There is absolutely no rush on your personal journey with energy healing. You are here, now, learning these techniques at exactly the right time, and it is precisely perfect for your unique life path.

Creating a sacred space around our energy prepares us for opening up our energetic fields. Through our conscious intention, we can direct the flow and shift the vibrational frequency of the energy in and around us. How we choose to "set the stage" energetically will directly affect how the rest of our session will flow. "Like attracts like" in matters of energy: If we start in a busy, stressed, or chaotic state, we will undoubtedly attract similar resonating frequencies to our experience in that moment. If we take our time to shift our energy and move ourselves into a calm, peaceful, receptive, and loving state, our following experiences will mirror that vibration.

To create an energetically safe, healing space all around us, we must shift and elevate our energy first. The first two shielding exercises are ways to shift your energy into a calmer, more receptive state. I recommend trying each method at separate times.

See how you feel during each exercise, and how you feel afterward. Find the method that works best for you and your personal energy, then start each of these exercises with that method. If you're having "one of those days" and can't seem to shake it, do some of the conscious breathing exercises (page 124), and then meditate in stillness for a bit. Sometimes, simply slowing down and taking five minutes of your time to return to a peaceful state can make a *world* of a difference. If this doesn't shift your mood, wait for another time when you're feeling less stressed or leave the practice for another time.

Never, ever practice energy healing when you are angry or upset, or in a negative or fearful space. Always, always, always take the time to elevate your frequency first— before opening up to any spiritual work.

During your journey with energy healing, you'll discover where your strengths and sensitivities lie. Certain methods may resonate with you, and others may not. While undergoing this process of deep healing, you will slowly remove the layers and layers of everything that isn't truly you, until the divine light intelligence of your true Soul energy shines through. In this process, many things can change, including your sensitivities, preferences, and likes and dislikes. Try returning to this foundational section every few months and check in to see whether an alternative method may resonate with you at a different stage of your journey.

Visualization

Most exercises in this section start off with visualization. This doesn't mean you must have 20/20 third eye vision. All you need is a *willingness* to be open to trying new things, along with your imagination. For example, if I ask you to close your eyes right now and picture a teddy bear, you can easily do that. Let's try it.

Close your eyes and picture a teddy bear. Hold that image in your mind for a few moments. If it's not already, can you make this a three-dimensional image? Can you spin it upside down, or turn it around to face the other way? Can you imagine it twenty feet away from you? Now can you bring it right next to you? Can you make it much larger than you? And now small enough to fit in your hand? Can you make it disappear? When you're ready, open your eyes.

Even though the teddy bear does not physically exist in your reality, it 100 percent existed in your etheric, or energetic, reality. Your creative mind is a powerful tool that can manifest things into existence in the energetic realms. Just because you cannot see something with your physical eyes doesn't mean it's not there.

We are multidimensional beings living in a multidimensional reality. Stretch your mind (and your senses) around what actually qualifies something as "real." Do you have to physically see it or touch it to prove that it's real? Can you see electricity or touch gas? Working with energy means you'll be working within the subtle metaphysical realms.

You use your conscious, focused intention to create and structure your energetic environment in and around you.

Initially, you may not clearly "see," "feel," "hear," or "sense" anything around you that is beyond the five basic physical senses. The visualizations may seem like a dull picture at first, instead of high-definition color. With time and effort, your sensitivity to this subtle light information will increase beyond just the physical realm, and you'll "see" firsthand just how real your creative mind is when it comes to working with your energy!

We'll begin by intentionally shifting and lifting the frequency of the energetic space in and around us. These techniques will begin to gently uplift your energy and create a strong force field all around you.

Exercise: Column of Healing Light

The column of healing light is high-vibrational golden energy that flows in from the twelfth dimension into the stellar chakra. This golden light acts as an amplifier and an energetic immune booster to the auric field. This is a great technique to use when you've been feeling tired or depleted and like you can use a strong, vibrant boost of energy.

After you have set up your space, you may light a candle or incense. Set your intention to lift and elevate your frequency.

Find a comfortable seated posture where the spine is erect yet supported, and where you can place your feet flat on the floor. The spine should be able to maintain its natural curves and the body should feel relaxed.

Take a moment to gently close your eyes and tune into your breathing. Notice how your body and your energy are feeling at this time. With conscious exhalations, release any worries or tensions out and away from the body.

Take deep belly breaths and allow your breath to find an even, gentle pace.

From here, bring your awareness about three feet above the top of your head. You can visualize a horizontal golden, glowing disk spinning in this region. This disk is made of pure golden light energy and is about the circumference of a Hula-Hoop.

Visualize beautiful, sparkling golden light shining down from this disk all around you—similar to a light beam or column. You may feel, see, or sense this energy all around you. This light is gently beaming down and surrounding your aura and your physical body. If using golden light feels too intense at this time, switch to a pearlescent white light with golden flecks in it instead.

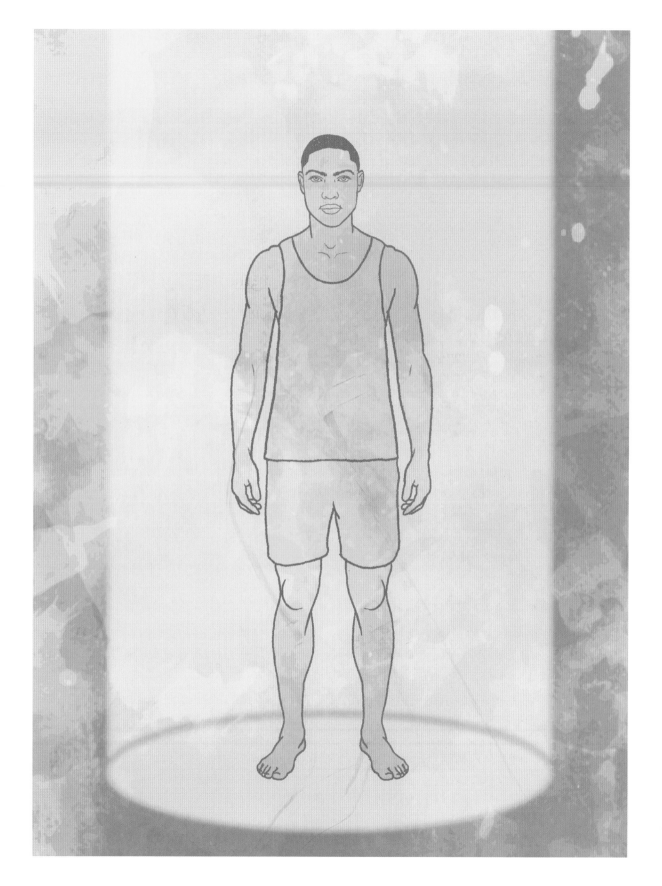

The intensity of the quality of light strengthens, as it begins to gently move down and into your crown chakra. Moving down and into the chakras, it permeates throughout the physical body, strengthening any areas of depletion and dissolving any areas of stagnant energy along the way.

You can adjust the "intensity" level of this healing light energy through your intention, lessening or amplifying the "saturation" according to what you need in this moment.

Take a few minutes to just sit and bathe in this energy as it is gently lifting your frequency, activating your chakras, and acting as a protective force field around you.

Once complete, gently deepen your breathing and visualize the light column softly disappearing around you, along with the golden floating disk it came from.

When you're ready, gently open your eyes. Take a moment to give thanks for the experience and then journal about it.

Exercise: White Bubble of Light

The white bubble of light is another high-dimensional tool to create a shield around you. This light typically does not come from outside of you, but it tends to come from activating your soul star chakra and expanding some of its light around you. This white light has a softer, gentler, more feminine energy to it than the golden light in the previous exercise, and is primarily used for purification and clearing. This technique is amazing to use when you feel energized but like you could use a quick clearing of your energy field.

After you have set up your space, you may light a candle or incense. Set your intention to lift and elevate your frequency.

Find a comfortable seated posture where the spine is erect yet supported, and where you can place your feet flat on the floor. The spine should be able to maintain its natural curves and the body should feel relaxed.

Now take a moment to gently close your eyes and tune into your breathing. Notice how your body and your energy are feeling at this time. With conscious exhalations, release any worries or tensions out and away from your body.

Take deep belly breaths and allow your breath to find an even, gentle pace.

From here visualize or simply imagine a giant bubble of white light forming all around you. It is emanating three to five feet all around you, in all directions.

This light feels soft, yet very protective. It allows you to feel the gentle and powerful vibration of pure Source light.

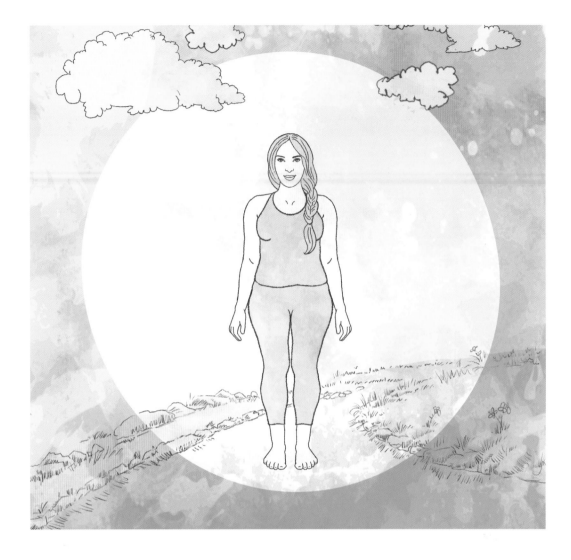

This light surrounds your auric field and physical body, and it also works on a cellular level, gently dissolving energetic impurities and disharmonious energies as it clarifies and amplifies your own light within. You may experience feelings of floating, bliss, or a lightness to your energy in this time.

Take a few minutes to just sit and bathe in this energy as it is gently lifting and purifying your frequency while acting as a protective force field around you.

Once complete, begin to gently deepen your breathing and visualize the white light bubble softly dissolving around you.

When you're ready, gently open your eyes. Take a moment to give thanks for the experience and then journal about it.

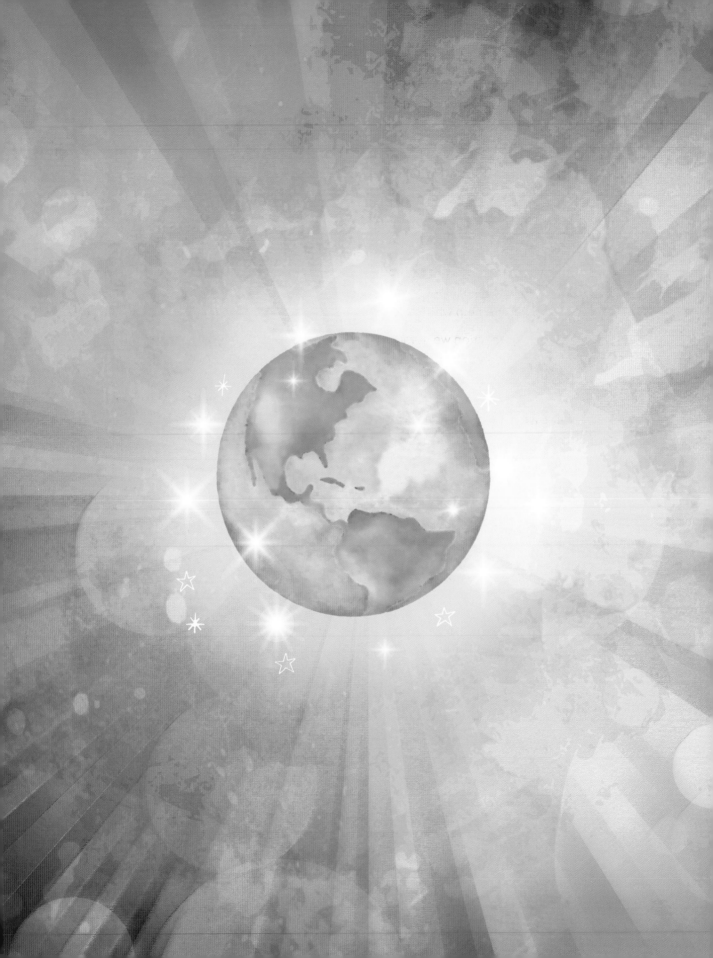

Grounding Your Energy

Grounding is a foundational technique used in many ancient shamanic practices. It's our energetic ability to connect with Mother Earth and receive her loving, healing frequencies to nourish, sooth, and replenish our energy field.

There have been many studies done on grounding, especially through the concept of "earthing," where it's been proven that when walking barefoot in nature for twenty minutes or more, there is definitive uptake of healing negative ions that flow up through your feet and into your body. Consistent exposure to these healing negative ions over time helps heal inflammation, clear free radicals, slow cellular oxidation, diminish pain, and help with anxiety and sleep issues.

This healing connection we humans have to the Earth has been proven scientifically, and has also been replicated through alternative medicine tools like "earthing mats" and "grounding wires." Through energy healing and the exercises you're about to experience, you will learn how to consciously create this energetic connection to Mother Earth from anywhere in the world, whether out in the country or fifteen floors up in a city building.

Consciously grounding and creating a connection with the energetic core of the Earth has many benefits. We can literally energetically "ground off," or release any excess or disharmonious energy from our fields. This can include excess emotional energy, excess mental or physical energy, and excess external energy we may have picked up from others during our day. The Earth uses these frequencies as compost, or fertilizer, as it ingeniously and effortlessly alchemizes and recycles these frequencies into healing light energy.

Once "grounded," we also can work with and draw up pure Earth energy, which can be experienced as nurturing, soothing, cooling, gravitationally heavy, slow, healing energy. Clairvoyantly, this is golden light, or occasionally green or terra-cotta colored sparkling light. The Earth's electromagnetic field has been measured at 7.83 hertz, also called the "Schumann resonance," after the physicist who discovered it in 1952. This is a very low and slow frequency that is similar to the theta brain wave frequency band, where deep and even miraculous healing can occur.

When consciously directed, Earth energy introduces its healing, slower frequency into our energetic system and physical body. This can stabilize our mood and promote a sense of deep relaxation, allowing the body's natural healing mechanisms to turn on. Earth energy creates a deep sense of feeling grounded and "at home" for many of those who have trouble sitting still in their bodies.

Many of my energy healing clients report a similar sensation to having a weighted blanket over them once they are filled with Earth energy.

Once a healing grounding circuit is created with this energy, it acts like a magnet for any disharmonious or disruptive frequencies in the body, gently pulling them down into the Earth for transmutation. Creating this grounding connection is wonderful for those who feel anxious, stressed, run-down, and ungrounded, or for those with nervous system disorders or sleeping issues.

Exercise: How to Ground Your Energy

Establishing an energetic grounding connection to the Earth comes easily to some and may take a lot of practice for others. Consistent daily practice will improve the quality, ease, and speed at which you can ground. Practice makes perfect, so give this a few tries, if needed, to get the hang of it.

Here are signs that indicate you have firmly established a grounding connection: feeling tingling or heaviness in the feet and legs or root chakra; a sense of deep relaxation; or, for most people initially, sleepiness. You also may see the golden light energy running through and circulating up the feet and legs during the process.

After you have set your space, you may light a candle or incense. Set your intention to create a grounding connection to the core of the Earth.

Find a comfortable seated posture where the spine is erect yet supported, and where you can place your feet flat on the floor. The spine should be able to maintain its natural curves and the body should feel relaxed.

Take a moment to gently close your eyes and tune into your breathing. Notice how your body and your energy are feeling at this time. With conscious exhalations, release any worries or tensions out and away from your body.

Take deep belly breaths and allow your breath to find an even, gentle pace.

Create a safe, energetic space by following the *Column of Healing Light* (page 94) or *Bubble of White Light* (page 96) exercise. Take a few moments to just "be" in this energy as it works to shift your frequency.

Once ready, bring your awareness to your lower back and the base of your spine, around the tailbone. Notice the heaviness of the pelvis and your seat on your chair.

Envision a golden cord or line of energy moving straight down from the tailbone, like a plumb line, toward the energetic core of the Earth with gravity's assistance.

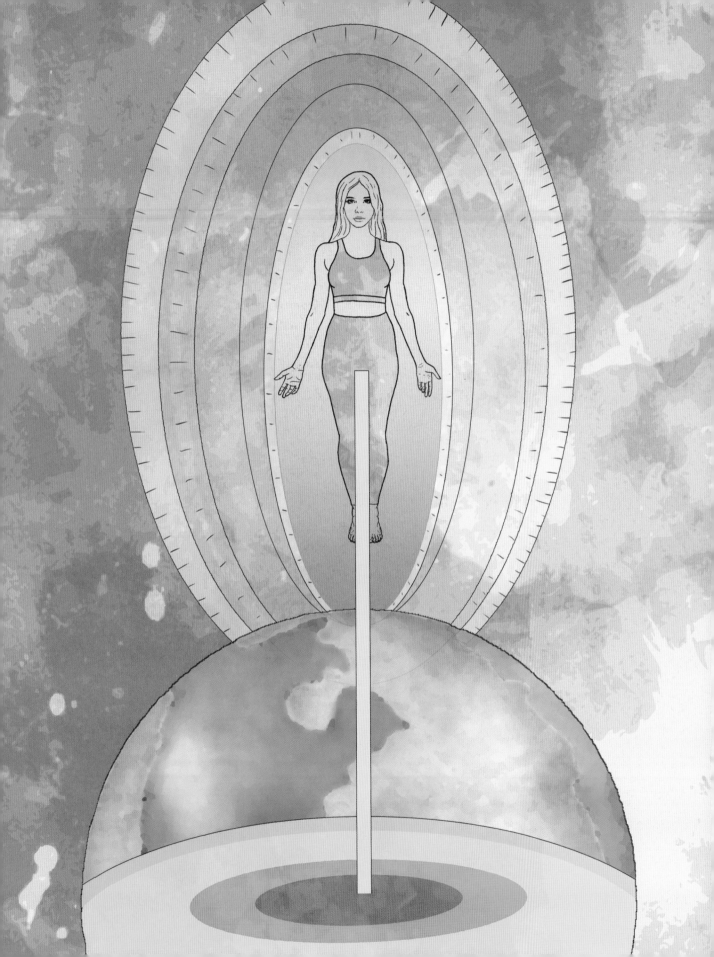

Visualize this cord moving past the ground floor, past the bedrock, past all the layers of the Earth, until it reaches and "links up" into the core of Gaia. Take as much time as needed to establish this connection.

From here, visualize a grounding symbol, such as roots or an anchor, to keep this cord connected in place. Intuitively go with any symbol that feels right for you.

Take a few moments to breathe here once you've established your first connection.

Now visualize the entire grounding cord expanding wider, maybe one to two feet in diameter. Breathe here as the connection grows stronger and deeper.

If you aren't sleepy, continue to the next exercise (below), keeping your grounding connection and column of healing light or white light bubble in place.

If this has been enough for this moment, keeping your cord connected, gently let the healing protective light around you dissolve by deepening your breath, and then gently open your eyes.

Take a moment to give thanks for the experience and journal the highlights of your energetic grounding experience.

Exercise: Bringing in Earth Energy

This exercise builds on the last one. Complete all of the steps to ground your energy (page 99). With your golden energy cord fully established and your protective light or energetic space all around you, you will begin to bring in the energy of the Earth.

With your grounding connection healing light established, expand your grounding cord to the width of your body. Take a few breaths as the connection deepens here.

Now open up your foot chakras fully and just breathe here as the Earth energy gently fills up your feet. The feet may feel tingly, electric, heavy—these are all good signs the Earth energy is flowing. Take a few breaths here.

Once the feet feel full of this Earth energy, visualize this Earth energy gently filling up and running up your legs, starting with the ankles and calves, then up to the knees and thighs, and eventually up to your pelvis and hips. Take as much time as needed to allow this Earth energy to circulate upward.

If visualization alone is challenging, you can add the use of your breathing to accelerate the process: as you breathe in, imagine that your inhale is drawing in and up the Earth energy. As you breathe out, the energy just remains and builds in that location.

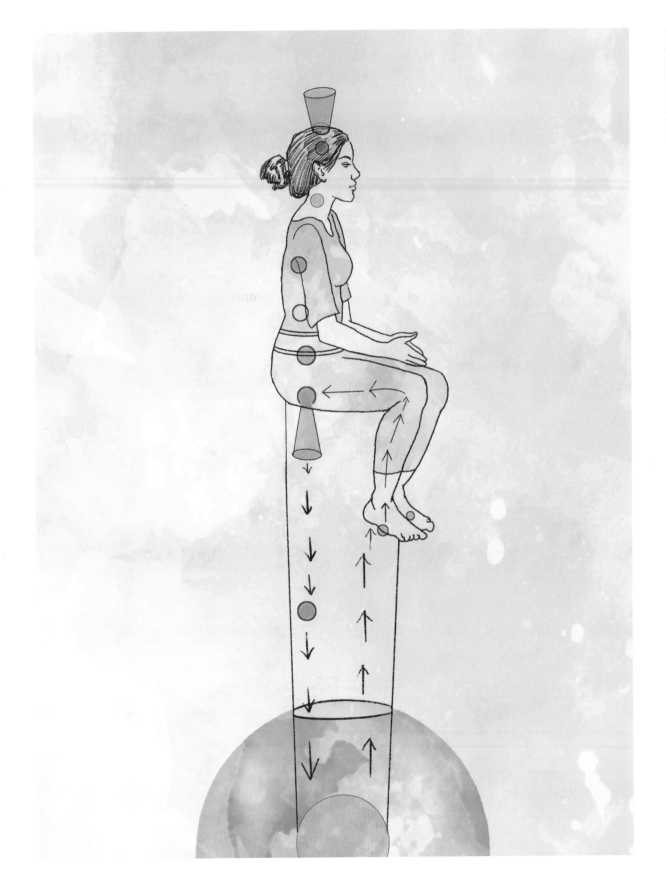

If you feel anxious, continue pulling up the Earth energy into your torso or any area of your body you feel needs this most, allowing it fill and gently soothe you.

Stay and meditate in stillness with this energy for a few minutes, allowing the body to adjust to this newer intensity of the Earth energy healing frequency. The energy is creating an even deeper sense of grounding with each conscious breath.

When ready, keeping your cord connected, and the circuit continuing, gently let your healing light column or white light bubble around you dissolve, by deepening your breath, and then gently open your eyes.

Take a moment to give thanks for the experience and journal the highlights of your experience. Did you get to subtly "feel," "sense," or "see" anything during the exercise? If not, don't worry; it can take some time initially. Rest if you need to so your body can fully integrate the healing effects of this newfound grounded connection.

Signs of a Grounding Connection

Here are physical and emotional signs that you have made the grounding connection:

- You feel calm, relaxed, and supported.
- You have a warm sensation of healthy circulation in your feet and legs.
- You feel firmly established in the present moment.
- You feel in the "flow" of life, and a loving connection to Mother Nature.
- You feel grounded and emotionally in a good place.

Here are physical and emotional signs that you are ungrounded:

- You feel off balance.
- You feel anxious, worried, or overly emotional.
- You're living in your head, repeating situations over and over again.
- You stub your toe or get in minor accidents a lot due to clumsiness from being energetically out of your body.
- You often lose your keys or can't find your phone or wallet.

Take inventory of how you feel after the exercise to see if you've made the connection or not. Also, now that you know this information, how do you feel you live daily? If you're leaning toward the signs that you're ungrounded, then practicing and mastering this technique is essential for you as a healer and will be highly beneficial for your overall state of well-being moving forward.

Alternate Grounding Techniques

Grounding is an important part of your energetic routine at the beginning of every session and to reestablish your grounding cord at the end of each session. This is an especially important technique to master before going into the more advanced exercises. Grounding can introduce you to a new way of being in your daily life, reduce anxiety, improve sleep, and help you remain calm in challenging or difficult situations. It is a practice I use daily, and before and after any meditation or healing work.

On a Soul level, we incarnated here in these physical human bodies, on this physical planet, to have this physical experience, as there is so much here to learn and so much beauty to experience in this life. If you have trouble accepting this, and have unconsciously kept your connection with Gaia closed, it is now time to explore why that was and work on reestablishing this loving and very innate relationship.

If you have experienced severe trauma, you are not alone: one in four Americans have. People who have experienced extreme trauma often have a tendency to energetically live "outside" of their own body. When this happens, grounding can feel nearly impossible. Remember that for all of us, energy healing work is a journey of self-exploration and discovery and an invitation for personal spiritual growth. This occurs first through awareness, and then through compassionately addressing and meeting these understandable, yet unhealthy, ways that we've energetically coped all our lives.

Your first priority is setting yourself up in the safest space available in your physical reality, before doing this work. Create very healthy boundaries around your time and your space. Next, it's about making your body energetically feel like a safe place to inhabit. You'll know in your heart if this information resonates with you. Follow the simple exercises in chapter 4 to retrain your nervous system. Practice the Earth grounding technique and then learn these exercises. Over time you will energetically fill your body with more and more light, making it feel like a wonderful, safe place to live.

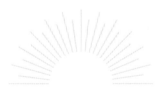

Initially, learning how to properly ground and actually maintain the connection can be challenging for most people. Try these additional techniques to assist you in making the connection a little bit easier:

- **Physically touch your body.** Move from your head, down to your shoulders, then arms, torso, legs, knees, and ankles, and then stay at the feet, adding light pressure until you feel fully back in your body.

- **Locate yourself in time and space.** State your name, along with the present time, date, and physical address you are located in (including which planet, seriously). This grounds your conscious energy back into the current time, space, and reality you reside in. This tool is simple yet effective! This is one of my favorite techniques to use, especially when I go on any meditation journeys or do any past-life healing work with clients.

- **Nourish your physical body.** Drink water or eat grounding foods such as root vegetables, cacao, and dark chocolate.

- **Do mundane chores.** Housework, such as cleaning your room, can help you be present and focus your attention on your current reality.

- **Go outside and get in nature!** Walking barefoot in nature and connecting with or sitting next to trees can be very helpful.

Working with Color Energy

Learning how to intuitively use colors to remedy issues can be helpful. Each color ray works on a different wavelength, or frequency band, and has its own speed, attributes, and resonance. You can learn to use color as an aid or healing tool, as an amplifier of energy, or as a way to cool down a situation.

Color energy therapy has been one of the simplest and most effective tools I've used in my practice. It can help clients boost their energy, vitality, and overall feeling of well-being in a short amount of time. When using color therapy in sessions, I never consciously pick the color for the client; instead, the color energy makes itself known intuitively and then I continue to hold that frequency and channel it into the client's auric field and/or chakra(s). Let's start with a few exercises that will experientially show you in an applied way.

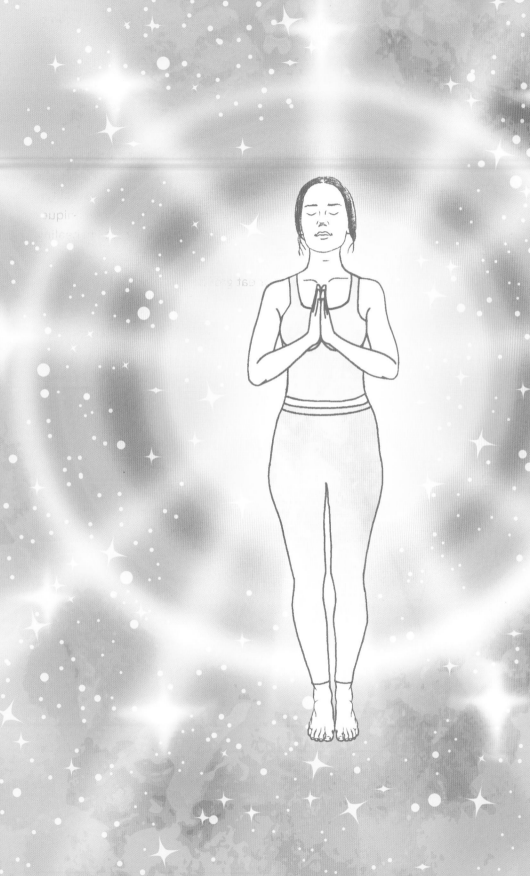

Exercise: Using Color to Boost Your Overall Energy

A note before beginning the exercise: When working with color energy, we always want the color to be clear, vibrant, shining, bright, translucent with a gemlike quality, and full of light. Colors with this nature can be healing and helpful when working with the chakras and auric field. Colors that are murky, dark, opaque, dull, or muddy will have the opposite effect.

After setting up your space, you may light a candle or incense. Set your intentions to intuitively work with color energy for healing.

Find a comfortable seated posture with your spine supported and feet flat on the floor.

Take a moment to gently close your eyes and tune into your breathing. Notice how your body and your energy are feeling at this time. With conscious exhalations, release any worries or tensions out and away from your body.

Take deep belly breaths and allow your breath to find an even, gentle pace.

Now take a moment to energetically create your safe, sacred space with either the healing light column or white light bubble technique (page 94 or 96). Take a few moments here to acclimate to the energy.

When you're ready, bring your attention to your seat and ground your energy through dropping a golden cord down to the core of the Earth. Once the connection is established, create roots or some anchoring symbol, so the connection stays strong. Take a few moments to breathe here.

Expand your grounding cord one to two feet or to the width of your body, and open your foot chakras. You have the option to circulate the Earth energy up your legs and down the root, down to the core of the Earth, or you can just breathe here with the grounding connection you've made. Either is great.

Now from here take a moment to tune into your body. Zoom out and take an intuitive overall picture of how you're feeling in this moment, with no judgment. Be neutral, as a simple matter of observation.

Now bring your awareness to about two feet above the top of your head, and intuitively ask yourself, "What color would be best to help boost my energy in this moment?" Go with the first color that came to your mind—whether it was an image, or you heard the color's name, or simply had a knowing, trust it.

Now visualize this color taking on a beautiful orb shape in this area two feet above your head. This color has a sparkling, shimmering, vibrant, and gemlike quality to it. The orb is about a foot in diameter and is spinning in place, fast. (To speed up the energy, I usually set it rotating directionally from right to left.)

This colored orb sprinkles some of its gemlike essence into your auric field, gently showering you with this color energy through every layer of the aura. It's filling up areas of depletion and remedying imbalances. Take a few moments here until the energy starts to subside on its own or when you feel intuitively that the process is complete—you'll get a thought, a nudge, or an inclination. Trust the subtle information you are receiving!

Now visualize bringing this color energy orb down and through your chakra system, starting at the crown chakra. Slowly pull this color orb through, and stop at each chakra point, noticing the effect of the color on your system.

When you're at the root chakra, allow the orb to move down into your grounding cord and gently dissolve there.

Take a moment to affirm your grounding cord connection, and when you're ready, allow the healing light column or white light bubble to disappear, and then gently open your eyes.

Take a moment to give thanks for the experience and journal about the color you used and your feelings around it, along with how each chakra responded.

Colors and Their Meanings

The color that is best suited for your healing practice one day might be completely different the next! Sometimes this can even shift by the hour. Our energy is constantly shifting with every thought, action, interaction, and response we take in our lives, and the color that intuitively came to you in the first moment is the one you needed the most.

By using your intuition, color can assist you and your current energetic state. Colors can charge the energy, cool things down, create focus, or provide healing. There is no right or wrong when it comes to intuitively using the beautiful, multispectrum, vibrant colors of the rainbow in your personal healing practice. Let's consider the energetic effects of certain colors and their meanings.

Colors and Their Applications When Working with Energy

Pink	Loving, nurturing, caring energy, soft, feminine (excess signals immaturity)
Red	Adds vitality, vigor, passion, heat, masculine (excess can lead to agitation)
Orange	Physical health and overall well-being, health of organs, leadership
Yellow	Joy, excitement, intellect, mental prowess, learning
Green	Enhances healing of all types, abundance
Light Blue	Calming, soothing, spiritual nature and thoughts
Royal Blue	The energy of truth, command, honesty
Indigo	Deep astral connection, third eye opening
Electric Blue	Can be an energetic anesthetic
Deep Purple	Royalty, respect, spiritual oneness, connecting with the Divine
Violet	Cleansing, purifying, very high vibrational and intense
Lavender	Soothing, spiritual, connects to the higher self
Silver	Abundance, purifying, feminine, can have a connection to ETs
Gold	Strengthening, fortifying, builds immunity, protection, healing
White	Source color, purity, healing, protection
Pearlescent Pastels	Very gentle, yet high, loving healing frequencies
Black	Atrophy, damage, death, deep despair or void energy
Brown	Muddied negative emotions or Earth energy
Gray	Anxiety, weakness, worries, neutrality

Exercise: Using Color Energy to Strengthen the Chakras

Here, we will use the traditional colors of the seven main chakras to boost and support each chakra individually.

Set up your space. Find a comfortable seated posture with your spine supported and feet flat on the floor. You may light a candle or incense. Set your intention to strengthen each chakra point.

Take a moment to gently close your eyes and tune into your breathing. Notice how your body and your energy are feeling.

Take deep belly breaths and allow your breath to find an even, gentle pace.

Now energetically create your safe, sacred space with either the healing light column or white light bubble technique (page 94 or 96). Take a few moments here to acclimate to the energy.

When you're ready, bring your attention to your seat and ground your energy through dropping a golden cord down to the core of the Earth. Once the connection is established, create roots or some anchoring symbol, so the connection stays strong. Take a few moments to breathe here.

Bring your awareness to your root chakra, at the base of your pelvis. Take a few moments to bring all of your conscious attention and awareness to this chakra. Now visualize a vibrant ruby red orb present in this area, filling up and boosting this chakra with its strengthening, sparkling light. Take a few minutes here and notice any visions, sensations, memories, emotions, or messages you may receive while connecting with this chakra.

Now move your awareness upward to your sacral chakra, below the navel. Take a few moments to bring all of your conscious attention and awareness to this chakra. Now visualize a vibrant orange orb present, filling up and boosting this chakra with its energizing, sparkling light. Take a few minutes here and notice any visions, sensations, memories, emotions, or messages you may receive while connecting with this chakra.

Move your awareness upward to your solar plexus chakra, below the ribs. Take a few moments to bring all of your conscious attention and awareness to this chakra. Now visualize a vibrant golden yellow orb present in this area, shining like the sun, filling up and boosting this chakra with its powerful solar-like light. Take a few minutes here and notice any visions, sensations, memories, emotions, or messages you may receive while connecting with this chakra.

Move your awareness upward to your heart chakra, located at the center of the chest. Take a few moments to bring all of your conscious attention and awareness to this chakra. Now visualize a vibrant emerald-green orb present, filling up and boosting this chakra with its healing light. Take a few breaths here and notice any visions, sensations, memories, emotions, or messages that you may receive while connecting with this chakra.

Move your awareness upward to your throat chakra, at the center of the neck. Take a few moments to bring all of your conscious attention and awareness to this chakra. Now visualize a vibrant blue orb present in this area, filling up and boosting this chakra with its truth-infused light. Take a few minutes here and notice any visions, sensations, memories, emotions, or messages you may receive while connecting with this chakra.

Move your awareness upward to your third eye chakra, located between the eyebrows, in the center of your head. Take a few moments to bring all of your conscious attention and awareness to this chakra. Now visualize a vibrant indigo orb present, filling up and boosting this chakra with its psychically charged light. Take a few minutes here and notice any visions, sensations, memories, emotions, or messages you may receive while connecting with this chakra.

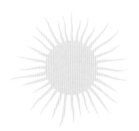

Last, bring your awareness upward to your crown chakra, located right above the head. Take a few moments to bring all of your conscious attention and awareness to this chakra. Now visualize a vibrant violet orb present, filling up and boosting this chakra with its spiritually purifying light. Take a few minutes here and notice any visions, sensations, memories, emotions, or messages you may receive while connecting with this chakra.

When ready, take a moment to reaffirm your grounding cord connection. Slowly allow the healing light column or white light bubble to disappear, and then gently open your eyes.

Take a moment to give thanks for the experience. Journal about the messages and information received and your feelings around working with each individual chakra.

You can also work intuitively with whichever color energy would work best for you each day. Following similar opening and closing steps, once in a meditative place, intuitively ask yourself, "What color would be best to help me boost my energy in this moment?"

Go with the first color that came to your mind—whether it was an image, or you heard the color's name, or simply had a knowing, trust that. Make sure the color is shining, transparent, and bright. Then visualize filling yourself up with this color, slowly, starting from the top of the head in a three-dimensional way, moving downward.

Envision infusing your entire physical body with the color energy, filling up every space, every cell, and every pore of your being with it, from top to bottom, like a French press. Once complete, sit with this energy for at least five to ten minutes, just letting it fully absorb and integrate into your system.

Outside of energy healing, you can bring more of this color energy into your life by simply wearing more of that color, eating more organic plant-based foods of that color, or using crystals in that color range. We usually do this intuitively without even consciously realizing the reason for it.

Sealing the Aura

Over the last few exercises, you've learned how important it is to start each session in a methodical and systematic way. Properly shifting your energy to a higher vibrational state and grounding your energy are foundational techniques for starting your energy healing sessions. As we dive into the deeper energy healing practices, learning how to properly "close down" and seal your energy after each session will be just as important.

In deeper energy work, our aura naturally opens up to channel and bring through healing energy and also allows blocked or negative energies to release. We do this when we open the energetic channels, heal and clear the chakras and aura, and even during "psychic surgery." In these cases, it is imperative to take the time to close and seal your auric field at the end of each working session.

Exercise: Closing Down and Sealing Your Auric Field

These simple steps are easy and quick, and will help make sure that the work that you've done remains safely contained so it can integrate into the physical system. "Closing down" also makes sure there are no "open doors" or windows in your energy field after your session. Here is an easy way to seal your auric field at the end of your sessions.

Set up your space and find a comfortable seated posture. You may light a candle or incense. Set your intention to learn how to properly close your auric field.

Take a moment to gently close your eyes and tune into your breathing. Notice how your body and your energy are feeling.

Take deep belly breaths and allow your breath to find an even, gentle pace.

Now energetically create your safe, sacred space with either the healing light column or white light bubble technique (page 94 or 96) and take a few moments here.

When you're ready, bring your attention to your seat and ground your energy through dropping a golden cord down to the core of the Earth. Once the connection is established, create roots or some anchoring symbol, so the connection stays strong. Take a few moments to breathe here.

Bring your awareness to the outer edge of your auric field. This is the seventh layer of the auric field, which is typically around an arm span away in every direction, or three to five feet in diameter. You can use your intuition to "know" where the edge of your aura is, ask for an image in your mind's eye to "see" the edge of your aura, or even use your hands to slowly "sense" its outer boundary.

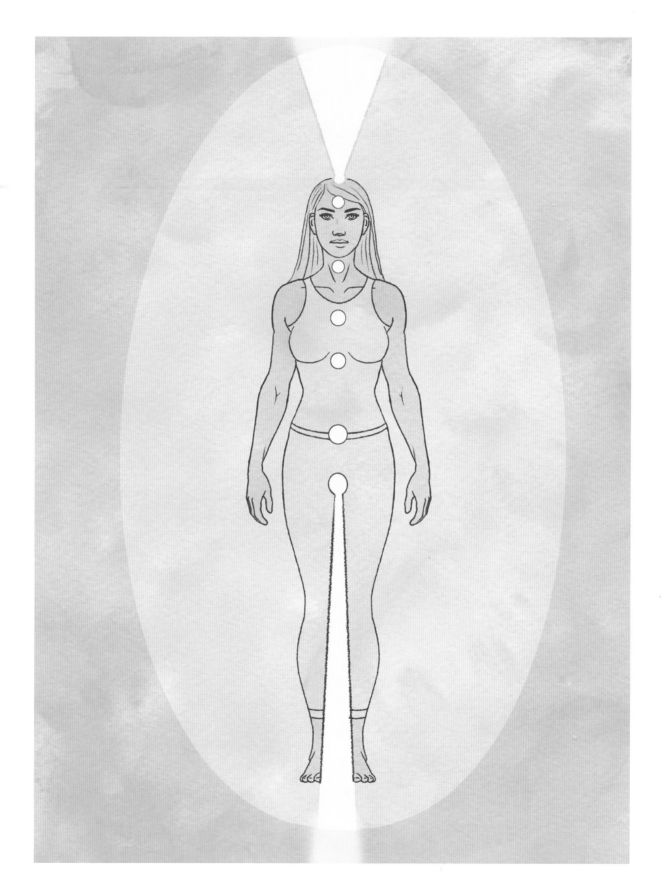

From here, to seal your auric field, visualize a golden layer of light all around the outermost layer of your aura. This light can be a hollow golden egg or a golden bubble. This can also look golden lines of light woven tightly together like mesh, or golden geometric patterns in an egg-like shape around you. Whichever image resonates with you most, use that.

Feel as if this light frequency has almost a solid quality to it, a hardness, as if it were physical.

To close your session, you have several options: You can verbally state, "This session is now complete!" You can visualize an open door closing shut or closing an open book (or anything of that nature) with the intention of sealing the session. You can also simply intend and mentally affirm that you are now closing the connection. All are effective methods for succinctly ending your session.

When ready, take a moment to reaffirm your grounding cord connection. Slowly allow the healing light column or white light bubble to disappear, and then gently open your eyes.

Take a moment to give thanks for the experience and journal about which closing methods worked best for you.

In this book, I may refer to the starting process of tuning into your breathing, creating your energetic safe space through either the healing light column or white light bubble, and grounding your energy as "setting yourself up energetically." I may also refer to the ending process of sealing the outer layer of your auric field with golden light and closing with a statement or image as "sealing and closing down."

The Best Protection Is a Full, Healthy Aura

Recently, some teachings have suggested putting up an energetic shield by using different colors to protect yourself—similar to how we just sealed our auras in the last exercise. Although, yes, adding an extra layer of light around you can help if you are feeling energetically vulnerable, I do want to clarify that it is a little bit like only mopping the floors without actually fixing the leak.

Our best form of energetic and psychic protection is a healthy, full, and intact auric field. This means:

- All layers, one through seven, are clear, vibrant, and healthy.
- The layers are full of energy.
- The layers have no depleted areas, rips, tears, or openings in them.

Keep in mind, these are essential elements, but there can be additional unseen or unaccounted for factors beyond this list. Working on healing and repairing the different layers of our multidimensional auric field is an advanced practice. It's one we will be going over only briefly toward the end of the exercises, but doing so can provide the amazing ability to feel (and remain) strong and full, from the inside out. A healthy, full aura acts like Teflon to any incoming lower vibrational frequencies: you are literally so energetically "full of yourself" (in a good way) that there is no room available for any outer intrusive energies to come in. Working on strengthening and filling in your auric field will grant you far superior protection than any light shield can, because it goes many layers deep.

Some signs that your aura is depleted are:

- You feel "at the whim" of everyone and everything around you.
- You feel sensitive to and bogged down by simple social interactions.
- You get colds and flus often.
- You feel the energies around you so strongly and feel like you "take them on" instead of neutrally observing or emitting your own frequency.

Doing the deep work of healing your auric field, which processes in layers and layers, will strengthen you as a healer. Regular practice of the exercises in this book will help lay the groundwork. Additionally, one of the quickest ways to boost your auric field is to bring in the frequency of divine love. This is not the romantic, dramatic, human version of "love." It is the sublime, blissful feeling of unconditional love for all beings, things, and experiences.

Bringing in this frequency of divine love, through practices like the gratitude meditation in chapter 4, and then maintaining it for as long as you can, will help strengthen each layer. This frequency also acts like a buffer, where the outside lower vibrational energies just dissolve as they meet your aura. This is a great tool to use along the way to completing your healing process and fully healing your auric field.

Practices to Increase Energetic Sensitivity

As you heal your energy, your extrasensory "gifts" will strengthen and open. Clairvoyance (clear seeing), clairsentience (clear feeling), clairaudience (clear hearing), and claircognizance (clear knowing) are just a few examples of the *many* amazing gifts we are all innately hardwired with. Every human has these abilities in their reach, but depending on many factors, these have either been shut down at an earlier age, gone dormant, or haven't been allowed to bloom and develop. (There are also possible karmic reasons due to past-life actions that can affect why some people's gifts may be turned on or off, but for this book, I will stick to this lifetime.)

Just because a person has their clairs turned on doesn't mean they're more gifted, talented, psychic, or capable than anyone else. It simply means that they've made it a priority and put time and effort into refining these abilities.

Developing and honing your gifts is an important part of the energy healing practice because it allows you to receive invaluable information about what's going on with your energetic field. This nuanced picture allows you to work directly with the issues at hand and helps you perform a more detailed and accurate session on yourself. Opening and training your extrasensory gifts will strengthen your skills as an energy healer and allow you to work with proficiency, confidence, and ease.

There are primarily two schools of thought on opening our psychic senses. Some believe that once a certain level of energetic work has been done, and spiritual maturity has been attained, your gifts will naturally open up. Others believe this is not the case, and that you must practice and put continuous effort into opening and strengthening your gifts for them to work. Knowing that anything is possible, I believe that it can be a combination of the above. To assist you in your healing journey, I've provided several exercises for you to practice developing your energetic sensitivity. These exercises are not a onetime thing and are meant to be practiced consistently until results are achieved. Learning to first work with your clair gifts is just like learning how to ride a bicycle: use these exercises as temporary training wheels to help you get started, and with practice and patience, you'll be on your way to riding solo!

Clairsentient Exercise: Activating the Palm Chakras

This exercise is all about gaining the ability to send healing energy through our hands—and then to use our hands as sensory tools when assessing our energy field and chakras. This is an extremely helpful way of working with energy. Many people find they are able to send energy through their hands in a much stronger and more precise way than simply working through visualization. The added benefit when working with the palm chakras is you can get a new sensory form of "feedback," which can feel very physical.

Set up your space and find a comfortable seated posture. You may light a candle or incense. Set your intention to activate your palm chakras before beginning the exercise.

Begin the step-by-step practices for "setting up energetically" now. These should be automatic but refer to previous exercises (pages 94 and 96), if needed.

Now bring your hands together in prayer pose and rub them firmly together for about a minute, quickly enough to generate heat and energy in the palm chakras. You can clap your hands a few times as well once this is done.

With your eyes remaining closed, keeping your hands in prayer position, bring your awareness to the heat generating inside your hands.

Now gently separate your hands about two inches apart, and with your eyes closed, keep all of your concentration and awareness between your hands. Consciously send your energy into this space. Take a few conscious breaths to do this.

When ready, slowly oscillate your hands, one inch closer together and one inch wider apart (the slower the better). See if you notice any sensations, pulsations, feeling of pressure, temperature changes, or tingles happening as you do this.

This work is very subtle at first, so if you do not "feel" anything yet, charge your hands up again by rubbing them together and try again, even more slowly this time.

For those of you who can distinctly feel the energy between your hands, visualize it forming into a tiny orb. You should be able to tangibly feel the sensation of pressure in your hands when you push inward toward the center. It feels similar to two magnets of the same charge pushing against one another.

From here, using your conscious awareness, focus on the orb and gently stretch and make it bigger, by slowly separating your hands about two inches wider apart, then gently push back only an inch to see if the orb is still intact and you still feel its outer boundaries.

If this was possible, then widen the orb another two to three inches apart, and again, push back gently to feel its boundaries.

Keep playing with this and seeing just how far you can expand the orb, while still maintaining the firm, tangible ability to "feel" the orb with your palm chakras.

If you lose the connection or become distracted, start over from the beginning by rubbing your hands together, and then continue. Ideally, you should be able to eventually separate your hands about one foot apart and be able to maintain the sensation of the energy orb in your hands.

If not, then follow the next few steps to close. Bring your awareness back into the room and reaffirm your grounding cord connection. Seal your aura and close your session, and then gently open your eyes.

Take a moment to give thanks for the experience and journal about the sensations that came up for you.

Clairvoyant Exercise: Practice Seeing Auras

For this next exercise, you can choose to "set yourself up energetically" or not. The reason I recommend doing this each time is because it raises your frequency, helps protect your energy, and heightens your intuitive senses. To prepare for this exercise, you'll need a white sheet of computer paper, a white, clean wall, and a partner or plant to practice with.

Part 1: Seeing Your Own Aura

Set up your space and find a comfortable seated posture. You may light a candle or incense. Set your intention to clairvoyantly "see" your own and your partner's aura before beginning the exercise.

You have the option of "setting yourself up energetically" now if you choose. From here, grab your sheet of paper and place it on a flat surface like a table or chair.

Rub your hands together to activate your hands. Now place one hand hovering a few inches off the paper, fingers spreading normally. Try to make sure there is no harsh shadow cast underneath you for the exercise. If so, adjust your lighting or position.

Soften your gaze and focus just above your middle finger. Don't try to strain your eyes to find a point on the paper, but instead, soften the focus of your eyes so everything is a little bit blurry. Continue to concentrate with your gaze here above the fingertips while keeping the gaze soft for as long as you can. Blink when needed but keep the eyes soft and the concentration above the fingers.

If you break focus, start over again.

Notice if you see any soft outline of light around the outer edge of the fingers and hand. If you do, don't avert your eyes, but instead, continue your steady, soft focus above the hand. The longer you're able to do this, the stronger the auric image may become. Bonus tip: Sometimes it can help to look through your peripheral vision if you're struggling with looking straight on.

If you've noticed a glowing outline, congratulations! You are typically seeing the first layer of the aura. I usually see this layer as an electric shade of blue.

If you can stay here longer, continue keeping your gaze soft and notice if other layers, further out from the first, appear. If not, that's all right; this takes time. When complete, journal what you saw and then continue back to the exercise.

Part 2: Seeing Your Partner's Aura

Now find your partner and ask them to sit in front of the white wall, with their back against the wall. If you can't find a partner, you can do this exercise with a plant instead. Sit four to five feet across from them.

Similar to your hand in the last part of the exercise, soften your gaze a few inches above your partner's head or above the top of the plant.

With your gaze remaining soft the whole time, continue to concentrate a few inches above their head for as long as you can. Blink when needed but keep the eyes soft and the concentration above their head or above the top of the plant. If you break focus, start over again.

Notice if you see any soft outline of light around the outer rim of their body. If you do, don't avert your eyes, but instead, continue your steady, soft focus above their head. The longer you're able to do this, the stronger the auric image may become.

Continue until you've seen the first layer of the aura: this may look like an afterimage at first, but it will develop into color with relaxed concentration.

If you're feeling ambitious, and your partner is patient, slowly lift your gaze just a few inches higher, holding the soft vision of your partner and the first layer of their aura. Sit for some time and see if another layer or color of their auric field appears. If not, that's all right; this takes time.

When you're ready, begin to "seal and close down" to end the experience.

Take a moment to give thanks to your partner and give thanks for the experience, and then journal about any image you may have seen around your partner or plant.

We usually have one (or occasionally two) very strong senses to start with. If one exercise was more successful than the other, then wonderful! You've discovered your primary sense. This isn't to say that you should lean on that area alone, but it *is* helpful to have at least one activated and strong clair sense for this work, and then eventually, over time, you can develop the others. Clairvoyance, along with all of the gifts, can take time to develop, so please be patient with yourself during this process.

If you've tried this exercise several times and have had no luck, then take a break and come back to it in a week with "fresh eyes," so to speak. Keep trying and know that working with your gifts can be similar to growing a seedling. Every time you practice these exercises with love and attention, it is like you are watering and nurturing that seed. Just because you haven't seen it sprouting above ground yet, doesn't mean that it's not growing or that monumental changes aren't taking place. It can be as simple as the first (insert hypothetical number) practices yielding no results, and then (hypothetical number) practices plus one, and success! The moral of the story is that you'll never know when the seed will sprout, so keep practicing with love, diligence, and patience.

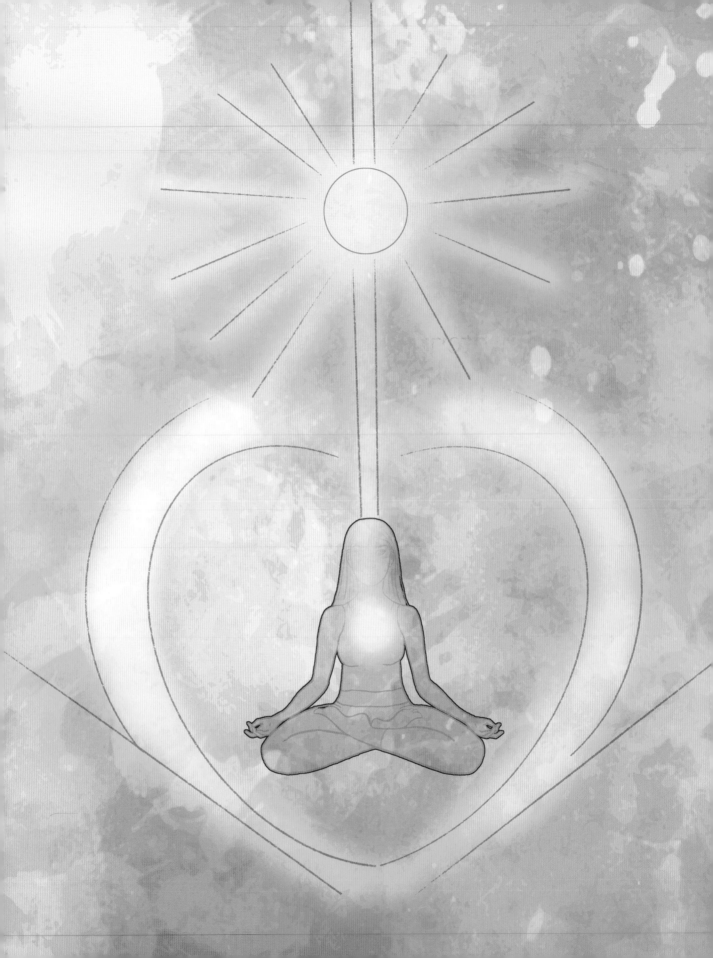

8

Intermediate Energy Healing Practices

●

Welcome to the intermediate level of your energy healing practice! This is a big step toward bringing in more of your Soul's light and learning how to regulate your own energy field. Make sure you've taken some time to get comfortable working with the exercises from the previous chapter, as we'll be building upon a fundamental understanding of each one.

This is a beautiful and exciting time for you. We'll be working on activating the proper energetic channels needed for hands-on healing. Sending healing energy through your hands is one of the most powerful and effective ways to amplify and direct the healing frequencies you're receiving. Your hands are also an amazing tool for scanning and discerning what's best needed for each of your personal energy healing sessions.

Opening the Channels

Through breathing exercises and meditations, you've been unconsciously clearing and healing your energetic channels. This simple process brings in so much fresh energy and light into the body and the energy field. The original purpose of these meditations was to allow you to drop into the feelings of peace and stillness for you to find ease and success with your energy healing practice.

The following guided exercises use our breathing and our intentions to move the energy in a particular way to fully activate our energetic channels. These channels are not physical, but you can think of them as mini tubes of light running through your system. They are similar to the yogic nadis and Chinese medicine meridians, but instead of working with one pathway at a time, imagine a symphony of beautiful harmonious pathways firing together to direct and send the healing currents to specific areas throughout the body.

In these exercises we will learn which primary pathways to use during energy healing to channel healing energy into the body and out from the hands. This is a sacred set of activations, so please treat it as such. Set up your space for the highest outcome before you begin.

Activation Through Intention with Conscious Breathing

The easiest and most potent way to channel healing energy for your practice combines these two practices: setting intentions and consciously directing your breathing. This differs from simple meditations where we become the observer, witnessing our breath flowing through us. These will (initially) be more active practices where we are intentionally directing the flow of energy through the body. We will activate the sacred energetic channels, so before each practice begins, please take the time to set up and clear your space, so only the highest frequencies are flowing around you.

Next, it's important to set the intention that you will now be consciously using your breathing to bring in and direct the energy's flow. The breathing works like this: As you inhale, you consciously intend and visualize pulling in healing light energy either through your crown chakra or your foot chakras into your heart chakra. As you exhale, you send out this healing energy from the palm chakras in your hands. Once you repeat this cycle consciously a few times in a row during your session, the energy begins to naturally follow in the direction you give it on its own.

When practicing energy healing, you may also send healing energy out from the heart chakra (or the other main seven chakras). For most people, their heart chakra (and additional chakras) usually need some emotional healing and energetic clearing *before* being able to properly do this, whereas the (very neutral) palm chakras (typically) do not. For most people, it's usually much easier to send energy through their palms than the seven main chakras, and it flows out much stronger and more succinctly too. When working on yourself at home, you will primarily use your hands as your main method of sending healing energy into the body, chakras, and energy field.

Before working on drawing healing energy *into* the body from the outside, it is very important to first make the connection *within* our own system. This will allow for the proper flow of energy to move throughout our system with intention. When the head and the heart are working together harmoniously, we operate from both the divine masculine aspect of logic and intellect and the divine feminine aspect of intuition and feeling.

Working out of balance with just one or the other can create issues with discernment, where we overthink everything, leading to inaction, or we act carelessly without upholding personal boundaries. When these aspects are disconnected or unintegrated, it can feel like a constant battle between mind and heart, leading to a lot of doubt around which decisions to make. When these aspects are integrated, there is a beautiful flow or dance of energy between the mind and the heart, allowing for our intuition to strengthen and work together with the proper discernment from the mind. This connection is essential when it comes to hearing and interpreting the best course of action within each energy healing practice session we do.

Exercise: Connecting Head to Heart

Begin this exercise with a short activation meditation to clear and strengthen the connection between the mind and the heart. These activation exercises will be a continuation from one another, so try to complete these three in a row. If that's impossible, or you become sleepy after one of them, then just relax and pace yourself. The entire activation will take around one hour, but you can break it up into twenty-minute periods each. If so, energetically set yourself up each time and close yourself down after each exercise.

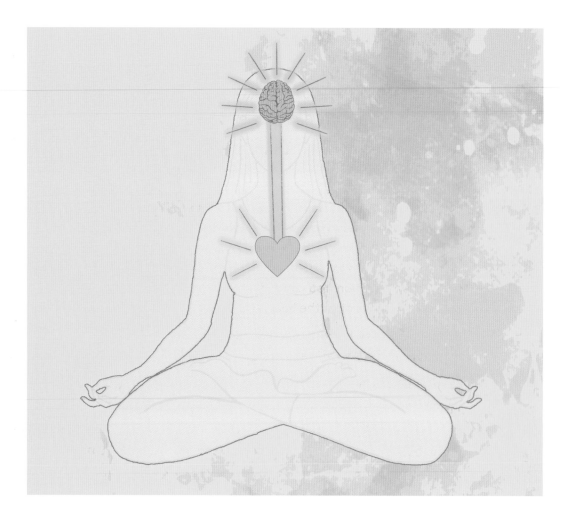

Set up your space and find a comfortable seated posture. You may light a candle or incense. Set your intention to clear, heal, and activate the connection between your mind and your heart.

Take a moment to gently close your eyes and tune into your breathing. Notice how your body and your energy are feeling.

Take deep belly breaths and allow your breath to find an even, gentle pace.

Now, energetically create your safe, sacred space with either the healing light column or white light bubble technique (page 94 or 96). Take a few moments here.

When you're ready, close your eyes, and bring your awareness to your third eye chakra in the center of your head and your heart chakra in the center of your chest. You can visualize these as glowing orbs of light in the centerline of your body, the heart being emerald green and the third eye being indigo.

Now bring your attention to the middle point between these two chakras, around the level of your collarbones. Visualize a small golden orb, about the size of a golf ball, appearing in this center point.

As you breathe in, visualize bringing this tiny golden ball of light vertically down a straight pathway to touch the heart chakra orb. As you breathe out, visualize the golden orb moving vertically upward on that pathway to reach and touch the third eye indigo orb. Do this slowly. As you breathe in, the orb travels down to the heart. As you breathe out, the orb travels up to the third eye. This is clearing and creating a strong connection between the two before the activation.

To make this practice stronger, place the first two fingers of your right hand on your third eye, and the first two fingers of your left hand on your heart chakra. Add *very slight* pressure with the intention of stimulating the chakras to strengthen their energetic connection. You can also use frankincense or sandalwood essential oils at the third eye and rose oil at the heart as a separate additional option.

Take a few slow, methodical breaths, visualizing this golden orb traveling up and down this pathway, clearing and strengthening the connection between these two points.

From here, you can release your fingers and take a moment to breathe, bringing the golden orb and your awareness back to the vertical center point in between these two points.

Now, set the intention that as you breathe in, this golden orb of light strengthens, and as you breathe out, this golden orb begins to slowly stretch vertically in both directions (only about an inch higher and lower with each exhale) to form a beautiful tiny tube of golden light. Each inhale strengthens the golden energy and with each exhale, the light tube extends vertically longer in each direction. Take this slowly, and keep using your breath to build and fortify this connection.

Once your golden tube has reached both chakra points and has solidified this connection, starting from the center, visualize breathing in pure white light through the inside of this tube in the same way. Each breath slowly continuously fills the tube a little bit more in both directions.

Once the white healing light has reached both chakra points, simply close your eyes and breathe. Remain here for a minute or two, concentrating on the connection that was made and observe whether you are receiving any messages or insight in the form of feelings, visions, hearing, or a knowing.

When you're ready, gently open your eyes, give thanks for this newly solidified energetic connection between the mind and the heart, and journal your experience and any insights.

Exercise: Crown to Palm Chakra Connection

The next two exercises will activate our ability to heal with our hands, also called "laying of hands." In both exercises, we will be pulling in high-vibrational healing frequencies directly from an external source into our bodies and then channeling them outward from our hands.

Take a moment to get comfortable once again. Set your intention to clear, heal, strengthen, and activate the energetic pathway from the crown chakra to the palm chakras.

If you choose, take a moment to call on the highest power of the divine consciousness, asking to fill, bless, and protect this activation with the frequencies of the highest love, light, and truth. You may also call on your higher self, your loving team of lifelong spirit guides, and archangel Michael to oversee and protect this session for you. And, as always, only practice what resonates with you.

Now, rub your hands together vigorously for about a minute until they are noticeably warm. From here, place your hands on your heart, gently close your eyes, and tune into your breathing. Take a few deep belly breaths and allow your breath to settle; notice the warmth emanating from your palms. After a few moments, release your hands on your lap facing upward.

Bring your awareness to your crown chakra. Intend and visualize your crown chakra beginning to dilatate open, like a lotus flower blooming. Take a moment to notice what this feels like in the body.

Now bring your awareness even higher, moving directly upward along the vertical power current, traveling upward toward your stellar chakra (halo-like portal) about three feet above the crown chakra. Visualize a stream of beautiful diamond solar light (which comes in directly from our star, the sun) filling up your stellar chakra and streaming down vertically into your crown chakra.

With your awareness, follow this diamond solar light stream down into your crown chakra and take a moment to breathe here as it activates and bathes this center with high-frequency light. This light will be continuously streaming throughout this entire activation. Although this light is high vibrational and strong, it should feel loving and peaceful.

Now, allow this diamond solar light to slowly stream down the vertical power current into the center of your third eye chakra. Follow this light stream down with your awareness until it settles in the center of the third eye and take a few moments to breathe here as it strengthens and clears this center.

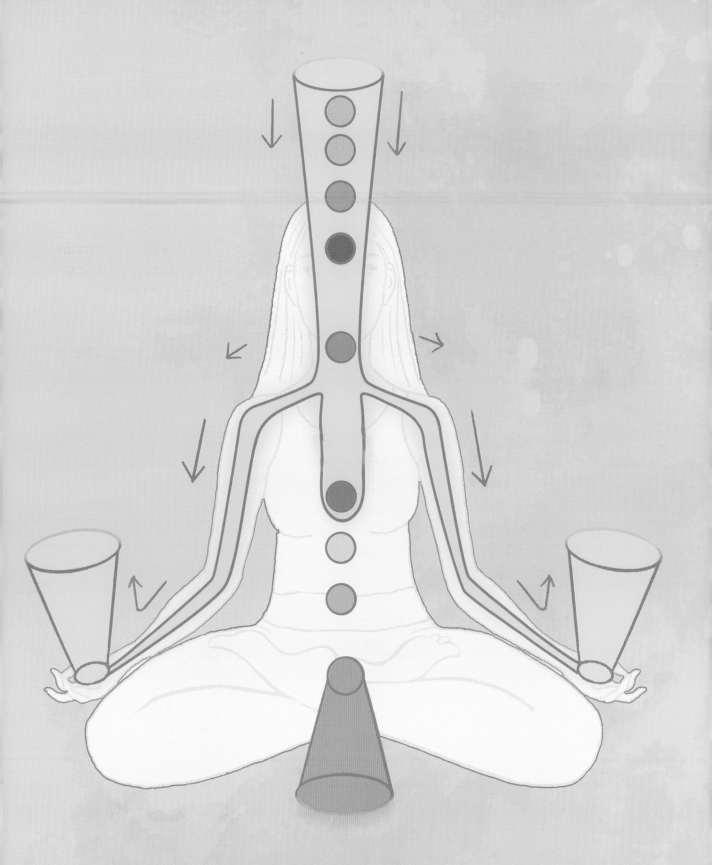

Next, let the light flow down your vertical power current into your throat chakra. Bring your awareness there and take a few breaths into this center to activate it. Now, let the light flow down the vertical power current into your heart chakra and take as long as you need here to allow this center to clear and activate.

Once your heart chakra is cleared and activated, guide this light back *up* the vertical power current to your throat chakra for a moment and breathe here. From there, allow this light to divide into two streams, running down your shoulders and into your arms, then to gently stream past the wrists and into the hands. Allow this light to fill up your hands to the point that they become warm or hot.

From here, bring your awareness to your palm chakras in the centers of your palms. Visualize these chakras dilating open to 100 percent of their circumference. Notice as the light gently streams out of your hands into your aura. You may notice this through seeing, feeling, sensing, or just a knowing this is occurring.

Now, consciously engage your breathing as a tool to fully activate this pathway: As you breathe in, intend and visualize consciously bringing in and down the frequency of the diamond solar light into your crown chakra and slowly down the vertical power current into your heart. As you exhale, move this light up the vertical power current into your throat, down your arms, and out of your palm chakras. Do this for several rounds, slowly and methodically.

From here, the connection has been established and this energetic pathway has been activated. Now all you have to do is simply inhale the beautiful diamond light down into your crown and exhale the light out from your palm chakras. Take a few rounds here to simply breathe and focus on this connection.

When ready, move your hands into your aura about two inches off the body, with the palm chakras facing inward toward the torso. Your palms can be facing your heart, throat, stomach, any organ, or any place you intuitively choose—go with the first place that comes to mind. Stay here with your hands in the aura for about a minute or two, just following the breathing connection, intentionally inhaling the light and exhaling it out from your palm chakras, now into that area of focus. Notice what you are feeling, sensing, or experiencing in the body at this time.

When you're ready, finish the session by bringing your hands together in prayer pose at the heart and thank yourself, along with all of the loving beings who assisted you in this activation, for this experience. Gently dilate your crown chakra back down to a comfortable circumference, and then gently open your eyes.

Take a moment to journal your experience from this activation.

This connection from the crown to the heart will always be with you. However, like any other skill, your ability and clarity with sending energy through this pathway will depend on how often you practice. When sending energy through your hands, it is primarily about setting the right intentions and then using your breath consciously to take in and then direct the healing frequency you're using.

This cosmic diamond solar healing light is one of the highest frequencies available to you, yet gentle enough to adjust to the individual. The more you practice working with this energy, the larger volume of light you'll be able to hold. When we start opening the channels, depending on how much of the preparation work and effort we put into our practice, we may only bring in 5 to 10 percent of the energy into our bodies at a time, without it being too overwhelming (you know it was if you fell asleep during your session). Eventually, with lots of time, practice, clearing, healing, and effort, we may hold and channel up to 75 to 85 percent of this light at a time. Some other beautiful frequencies you can use are those of divine love, peace, or the golden Christ light, along with individual frequencies from the beautiful rainbow spectrum of color light that we have been working with.

Be sure to practice working with one frequency at a time for a few practice rounds until you get *very used* to the energy and know what it *feels like* in your physical body. The more you work with a particular frequency, the easier it will be to hold this energy. After a few days (or weeks) of working with and strongly familiarizing yourself with one energy, then you can move on to the next. Move slowly with this practice and take time between working with new frequencies so you don't overwhelm (or "fry") your system's circuits. It's better to hold 85 percent of a particular light and strengthen your channels, as opposed to 5 percent of a bunch of random energies. When channeling energy, the experience should always feel relaxed, peaceful, and loving—and this depends on the energetic state YOU begin with and maintain throughout the exercise, not necessarily the frequency you're working with. If you do not feel relaxed, peaceful, and loving from the start, then wait until another time, when you are.

Exercise: Foot to Palm Chakras Connection

Next, we will be working with and bringing in the energy of the Earth (Mother Gaia) through our systems. You are already so familiar with this frequency, but now we will be using it in a different way, activating this energy for healing.

Take a moment to get comfortable once again. Set your intention to clear, heal, strengthen, and activate the energetic pathway from the earth star and foot chakras up to the palm chakras.

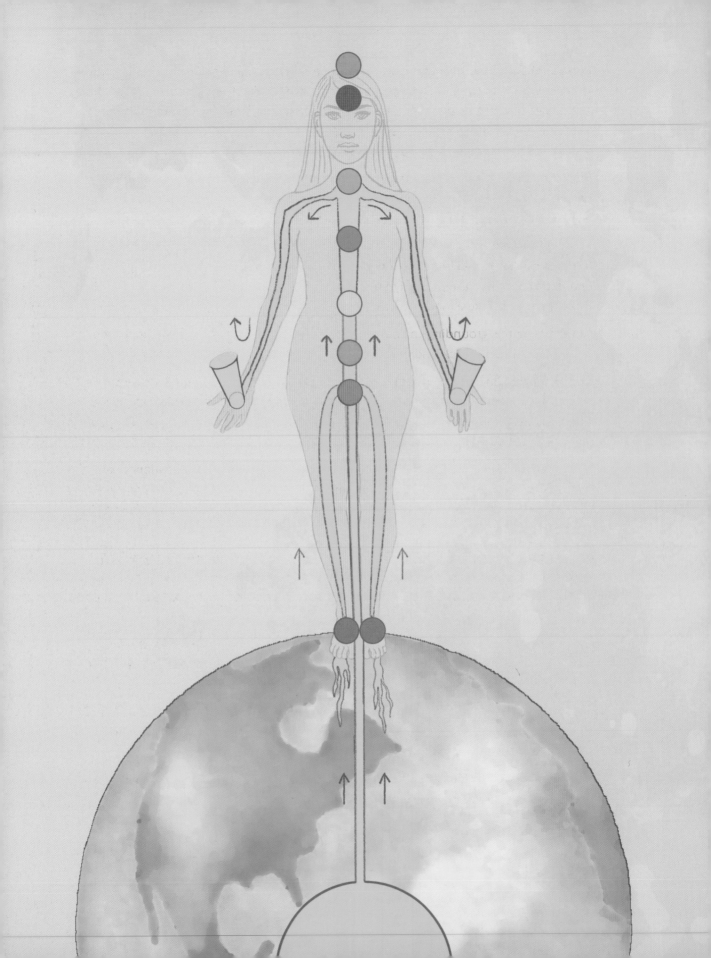

Rub your hands together vigorously for about a minute until they are noticeably warm. Then let your palms rest on your thighs facing down. Then rub your feet on the carpet or ground for a minute or gently massage the soles of your feet to activate them. (Is this necessary? No. Will it tremendously help the activation? Yes.)

Tune into your breathing and bring your awareness to your root chakra. Ground by intending and visualizing a golden line of energy extending down from your root chakra. Let it flow down into your earth star chakra (about two feet below your feet) and take a moment to breathe here, allowing the golden light to activate this chakra.

From here, continue extending this cord down from the earth star, past the different layers of the Earth, and let it connect directly into the seventh dimensional golden energetic core of Gaia. Optionally, you can visualize roots or an anchor to help stabilize this connection. Take a moment here to just breathe as you establish this connection.

Now, expand this grounding cord, growing it as wide as your physical body—in front of the feet, behind the back, and on the side of your hips. Take a few moments here.

Bring your awareness to your foot chakras on the centers of the soles of your feet. Dilate these chakras open 100 percent. You may already feel your feet start to gently tingle or pulse from the nourishing seventh dimensional Earth frequency traveling up your grounding cord connection.

Just breathe here as the Earth frequency gently fills up your feet. This frequency can sometimes feel cooling, slow, like gentle tingles, or even heavy, almost similar to the sensation of putting on a weighted blanket. This energy will be continuously flowing in from this point forward.

Now direct and intend that the energy flows upward and fills up the entirety of both legs—moving slowly from the ankles to the knees, the thighs, and eventually the hips and pelvis. Allow the Earth frequency to move into your root chakra and gently dilate the root open. Breathe here for a moment.

Guide and intend the Earth frequency to move upward along the VPC from the root chakra into the sacral chakra and breathe for a moment and notice what this feels like. Then, guide and intend this frequency continuously and *slowly* moves up the VPC to the throat chakra, stopping for a minute at each chakra and breathing.

From here, allow the earth energy to fill up and flow down into your arms, moving down into the hands. Allow this energy to fill up the hands until they feel full.

Dilate open the palm chakras to 100 percent, and allow the Earth energy to gently flow out of your hands and down into the legs for a moment.

Now, let's intentionally use our breathing to channel in this energy and move it through this pathway. Inhale, bring the Earth frequency up through the feet into the legs, exhale and let it build. Inhale, bring the energy up into the root and pelvis, exhale and let it build again. Inhale, bring the energy up from the root, into the vertical power current, traveling upward to the heart chakra, then exhale and let it strengthen. Inhale, bring it up to the throat and down the arms, then exhale gently and send the energy out from your palm chakras. Repeat this once more.

Now the circuit has been established permanently. Using your breathing, simply visualize and intend to pull in Earth frequency up through the feet into the heart as you inhale, exhaling from the throat chakra down the arms and out of the palm chakras. Your inhalation pulls the energy up through the feet, and your exhalation sends the energy out from the hands.

Now intuit a place on the body you'd like to send this Earth energy to and place your palms on that location. Take a few moments, consciously breathing and channeling the Earth frequency to this location: Inhale up through the feet, and exhale out of the hands into the body. Be fully aware of the sensations you may be experiencing, sensing, or feeling in the body at this time.

When you're ready, bring your hands together in prayer pose at the heart, and thank yourself and Gaia for this experience. Visualize sealing the outer layer of your aura with a layer or an egg of golden light, slowly dissolve your large golden light column or white light bubble, and then gently open your eyes. You can leave your grounding cord in place for the remainder of your day so Earth frequency can continuously flow in.

Take a moment to journal your experience from this activation. How was this different from the crown/diamond solar light activation? Did you have a preference working with one channel or frequency over the other? Why?

This pathway has now been established and the ability to channel in the frequency through your hands has been made. The more energy healing you do and the more you work with these frequencies, the stronger the energy will flow through the body and your system. Setting the intention for healing from the place of your heart and starting in an easy relaxed state of being will allow for the highest level of success while working with channeling in and sending out energy from the hands.

I want to congratulate you as you have just made and established the beautiful connection to the Divine and balanced frequencies of the "Heavens" and the "Earth." Working with these two frequencies alone on a consistent basis can bring unbelievable healing into your life. This is an amazing connection that is now permanently established, and it's up to you to decide what to do with it.

Experiment with the last two exercises by setting aside ten to fifteen minutes, picking which frequency and pathway to work with (diamond solar through the crown or Earth frequency through the feet), and then begin intuitively placing your hands in your aura or on different places on the body that you feel need healing and see what you experience. Use just one pathway at a time per session for the first few weeks (or months). Spend as much or as little time as needed in each individual area you intuit could use healing. When you feel complete with one area, move on to the next.

In a self-guided intuitive session, you may work with several areas or just one the whole time. Every day can be a different experience (or you may find consistent patterns). Be open to the experience. You can also work with one chakra or all the chakras—or the individual organs or muscle groups, depending on what you need. This is a totally customizable practice. If you have trouble intuiting what to work on, just start with your chakras from root to crown, or you can call in your higher self and ask them for guidance. There is no right or wrong formula for where to send your energy in these sessions, as *we are our own best healers*!

Always remember to set up your space and energy beforehand and seal off and close your energy afterward. Once you've become used to channeling in the energy in your self-guided sessions for a few weeks continuously, then extend the time of your sessions. Eventually, you can expand your sessions up to forty-five to sixty minutes at a time. If you get tired, get agitated, feel restless, or fall asleep during your session, then you've gone too long. Simply reduce the time for a few weeks until the physical body can acclimate to this new level of light. Give yourself time to rest and integrate these shifts in your body after each session.

Initially, practicing on yourself two or three times a week for a short period may be perfect. In the future, working daily for longer periods may work for you. Again, take your time and pace yourself, as you want to be very careful that you do not overdo it. Overdoing it and not resting or taking time in between your sessions in the beginning can have harmful effects at times, so pace yourself and allow your higher self and your physical body to assist you with messages along the way. It's very common during these sessions to experience some sensations described earlier in the book. Crying, tingling, sensations of warmth or cold, dreamlike visions or memories surfacing, and the feeling of deep peace are all common sensations that arise. Not experiencing these sensations but still feeling relaxed, better, or "lighter" after your session is a good indicator that it is working as well!

With energy healing, as in life, it is not necessarily about having the natural ability to do these practices, but it is instead about practicing with conscious intention to improve your skill. Initially, it is very normal to have a lower sensitivity in your body and palm chakras. But as you move along with your practice, the sensations and knowing will become stronger and stronger with each session, until you *know, without a doubt*, that the energy channeling through you is *real* and this process is flowing beautifully for you. Feeling a deeper sense of relaxation or peace after a self-guided practice session is a beautiful sign that it's working.

Working with a Pendulum

Tools can assist us with getting a clear picture of what's going on in our energy field and chakras. A pendulum is an amazing divination tool that works with sensing energy movement and vibration to gather information. We can use a pendulum in our energy healing journey to strengthen our intuition and, with practice over time, to assess the health and spin of the chakras. Originally, pendulums were used for locating water within land. In some Eastern countries, it's traditional to use a pendulum to determine the sex of babies before birth. When used properly, a pendulum can be a wonderful tool to assist you with gaining answers about your current energetic state.

Tips for Working with Your Pendulum

Pendulums are primarily used for answering "yes or no" questions and can be amazingly accurate when programmed and used appropriately with care. Working with a pendulum is a form of channeling. You should be in a positive energetic state when using it, and make certain that your pendulum is cleared properly after each use. Most pendulum pieces are made with crystal and you can follow a very similar protocol for clearing and programming them for use. Your pendulum can be programmed to gain answers from your higher self and can greatly accelerate your ascension path by assisting with the answers to many of your questions. A pendulum can also be influenced by lower vibrations, including your own desires, negative or fearful emotions, and outside energies around it. Working with a pendulum in this way, also called "dowsing," is a sacred art form and should be practiced with the utmost care and respect.

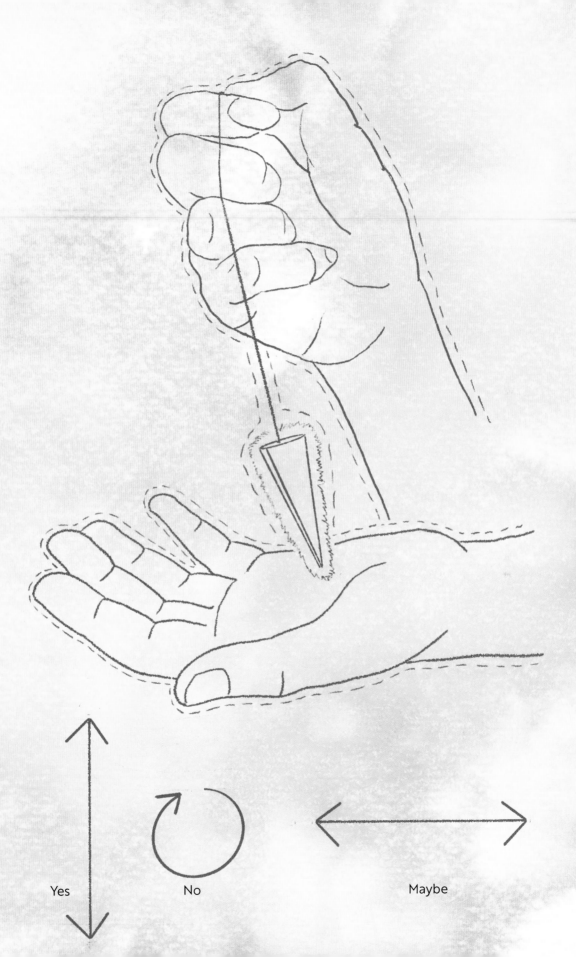

Yes   No   Maybe

To receive accurate answers, first make sure your energy is clear, your environment is clear, and your intentions are pure. Only embark on working with a pendulum if you intend to receive and know the Truth (and I mean the divine Truth with a capital *T*). It wouldn't be in your best interest to work with a pendulum if you're just looking for an egoic confirmation of your own opinions. A serious level of responsibility comes with opening up to Spirit in this capacity, so take honest inventory of how you feel inside before moving forward.

To receive accurate answers, you must be able to make sure that you are emotionally neutral on the topic you are asking about. If there is a strong desire or an emotional attachment to a particular response, then it would be in your best interest to wait to ask the question until you've neutralized your charge around it. Your emotional energy, if not managed properly, will strongly influence the outcome of your answer and increase the potential for inaccuracy. Setting up your energy and space, properly programming your pendulum, and remaining neutral around your questions are your three keys for success. Separately, it's important to note that pendulums do *not* predict future outcomes or events, as the "future" can always change at any moment.

Exercise: Clearing, Programing, and Testing Your Pendulum

Before using your pendulum, it's always important to clear it of any prior energies. I like to use a method taught by Dr. Marcel Vogel called "forced breathing," where through a powerful exhale, you strongly send your energy down into your palm chakra and into the crystal, programming it with whatever intention you've set before exhaling.

Hold your pendulum in your dominant hand and set your intention to completely clear your pendulum from all prior energies and programs. With a strong, quick, powerful exhale, send that intention into the crystal pendulum. Usually, this exhale method is done on every facet of the crystal, but with intention, it can work on the pendulum as a whole. The clearing may work on the first try, or it may take several tries, depending on the strength of your energy and your intention, so use your intuition as to when you feel it's clear.

Once your pendulum is clear, it's time to program it in a similar way.

Continue holding your pendulum in your dominant hand and, with loving intention, state out loud: "I now infuse this pendulum with the energy of divine Truth and love, with the intention that this pendulum illuminates the light of the Truth, and Truth alone." You can use this statement or something like it, with divine love in your heart and the emphasis on receiving the Truth.

Now hold the top part of the chain of your pendulum with your dominant hand, letting the main crystal piece dangle over the center of your nondominant hand, which is held flat underneath. To program its movements, sway your pendulum vertically in a line and tell your pendulum, "This movement is a 'Yes.'" Then have it stop, and move it in a circular motion and say, "This movement is a 'No.'" (Choose a different set of movements for your answers, if you'd like. What matters most is having the consistency of the programmed movement to its programmed response.)

When you have cleared and programmed your pendulums, it's time to test it. Ask simple "yes or no" questions you already know the answer to. For example: "Is today (insert correct day of week)?" "Is today (insert incorrect day)?" Or "Is my first name _____ ?" or "Is my pet's name _____ ?"

Occasionally, your pendulum may shake, which simply means it is searching for the correct answer. Once you have received all correct answers, then you are ready to use your pendulum!

It's always helpful to ground and center your energy or say a quick prayer for Truth before each use of your pendulum. It's also helpful to quickly clear your pendulum after each question session.

If your pendulum does not move at first, don't worry, it can take time. If that's the case, I recommend "setting yourself up energetically" and activating your palm chakras. This should assist you with getting clear, distinctive movements.

If you aren't receiving correct answers, then try clearing and reprogramming your pendulum again. If it's still not working, then it may be important for you to clear your own personal energy first, grounding off some of your excess emotional energy and clearing your physical space around you. You can also make a strong declaration: "Only energies that support the divine Truth are allowed here!" This will help clear the air around you and assist you in receiving accurate answers.

Enjoy your time working with your pendulum and remember, this is a *tool* for your spiritual and energetic development, not a crutch. Use it as an instrument to assist your intuition, where you use your intuition *first*, and then check your accuracy *after*, not the other way around.

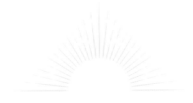

Exercise: Assessing Your Chakras with a Pendulum

Once you have become familiar with working with your pendulum, and you're skilled at receiving accurate answers, then it's time to take your dowsing practice to a new level! If you're still having trouble with the pendulum moving or the answers not being correct, clear and strengthen your energetic field first. Then wait a few weeks before trying again.

Dowsing is not for everyone, but it can be a helpful tool when it comes to quickly assessing the health and speed of chakras and energy, without having to clairvoyantly "see" or go into a deep meditation to do so. The pendulum can be used to get a "scaled" version of what is going on with your chakras. The pendulum can be trained to mimic the size and spin (or lack thereof) of the chakras to give you a clear idea about what is going on with your energy field. It will just take a session to program your pendulum to do this. Refer to the chart on page 142 to learn the movements and their corresponding meanings. This exercise can take from five to thirty, depending on the speed at which you and your pendulum can pick up the movements.

Take a moment to ground and center yourself by taking a few deep breaths. Set your space energetically the same way you've been doing in all of your previous energy practices.

Following the general steps from the previous exercise, using your breathing to "clear" the pendulum of all lower vibrations before beginning. (I like to do this each time I use my pendulum.) From here, communicate to your pendulum that you will be programming it with an additional set of new instructions.

When ready, take a look at the chart on page 142 and repeat the actions. So, for example, tell your pendulum to spin in a clockwise circle, and that this means a healthy, open chakra. It could take a minute, but the pendulum should move all on its own. If it doesn't, you can try moving it in that same direction and let it know what it means. Before moving to the next "action," make sure that your pendulum has accepted the program: ask it to show you what a healthy chakra looks like. Wait to move forward with each step until your pendulum can reproduce the proper corresponding movement with the correct command.

Once you have gone through teaching your pendulum these new movements and meanings and the pendulum has accepted the programming, then it's time to assess your own chakras.

With your pendulum hanging still and ready over your nondominant hand, ask your pendulum to show you your root chakra. Stay absolutely still as you allow the pendulum itself to respond and move on its own. Notice if your root chakra looks small or big, open or blocked, balanced or imbalanced between the masculine and feminine energies, and notice its speed. Without judgment, just observe what you see. When you have your clear answer, move on to the next chakra. Keep doing this until you have completed your assessment for the seven main chakras and then take down notes of what you discovered.

You can use this method as often as you need to assess the health of the chakras. After you have gotten familiar with this method, you can dowse the overall health of the chakra, and the individual fronts and backs of each chakra running along the vertical power current as well. With daily practice, you'll notice whether there are any patterns in your energy day to day. For example, are your chakras balanced and happily open? Are just the upper chakras open and not the lower? I call this pattern being "top heavy," which would tell me you need to incorporate more grounding practices. Are the lower chakras open but the upper ones are closed? This would be "bottom heavy," which would mean you can use some heart healing and meditation to clear your upper chakras. Is the crown way too open and the rest of the chakras are normal? This would show that the person tends to daydream often and leave their body energetically to escape reality.

We always want our chakras to be healthy and open. They should be moderately open, not enormous, as this can cause issues with "information" overload and a lack of boundaries. They should also be spinning at a healthy pace, not too slow, not too fast. We want the chakras to be balanced and not top or bottom heavy, but even and balanced compared to one another.

There are as many combinations of different energy patterns as there are humans on this Earth (or more!). The best way to interpret these meanings for yourself is to study the seven chakras in depth (see page 30) so you can understand what it means when a chakra is undercharged, slow, and depleted versus balanced or overcharged.

From here, you can form a picture of the common energetic patterns *you* may be holding in your daily living and assess what needs to be healed in the energy. This is a means of performing a short and simple energetic assessment on *yourself*, and *is not* a means to diagnose yourself or anyone else with any medical or psychological ailments or issues. The practice of dowsing is an art form and a skill that can take even the most intuitively gifted practitioners years of practice to develop.

Pendulum Movements & Meanings

(Inspired by Barbara Brennan's "Hands of Light.")

 Healthy, balanced chakra

 Unhealthy, closed, underactive chakra

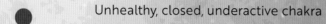 Blocked, stuck in physical perception

 Blocked, only spiritual perception, no action

 Feminine/yin energy overactive

 Masculine/yang energy overactive

 Too open, overactive chakra

 Chakra changing and shifting

Clearing and Balancing the Chakras

Energy blocks can be pockets or compiled figures of discordant and disharmonious energy. These are usually created from stored trauma responses or lower vibrational emotions being held or repressed within the energy. Blocks can happen consciously or unconsciously. They can also be caused by negative belief systems and ideologies that literally lead one to feel "blocked" in their life. Usually (but not always) the longer the belief is held, the longer it may take to release it or to physically heal from the changes during the integration period. The more acute, less "dense" blocks tend to clear much more quickly.

In a later exercise, we learn how to locate, clear, and release deeply lodged blocks and heal the energy around them. For now, let's work on a general clearing of the chakras. Practice this first before going in for the deeper, long-rooted blocks, as healing happens in layers. We don't want to overwhelm the system.

How to Clear a Chakra

There are different ways to clear, heal, and balance your chakras. When clearing lower energies from a chakra, the process typically goes as follows:

1. Identify the issue.

2. Gently dilate open the chakra.

3. Clear the chakra from the "inside out" (back to front) or from the "outside in" (front to back).

4. "Charge" or boost the area that has been cleared.

When working with a small, slow, or depleted chakra, you might need to take extra time to charge and boost the chakra to return it to its healthy state.

It will help to dowse and use your pendulum before these exercises to make your initial assessment, and then once more at the end to see whether your energy "work" is complete. However, dowsing is only one method of assessment. You can also use your hands (palm chakras) to "scan" your chakras and "feel" whether there are any imbalances (we'll discuss this is in more detail on page 145). If your clairvoyance is developed, you can view or "see" which chakras need clearing or healing. They may look darker or muddy, or have patches of darker energy, or lack vibrancy in their color. Another option is to go into meditation and simply work with your intuition to guide you, which may come in as a "knowing" around what chakras need healing.

Exercise: Chakra Healing with Gold Energy from the Inside Out

Here we will be learning how to bring in and send out high-vibrational energy in order to clear and transmute the denser, heavier, disharmonious frequencies from our system. This approach is also a wonderful way to charge and bring energy into the body, the first layer of the aura, and the chakras.

Set up your space and find a comfortable seated posture. Set your intention to clear, heal, and balance your chakras.

Take a moment to gently close your eyes and meditate. Bring in your healing light column or white light bubble (page 94 or 96) before beginning.

Now, bring your awareness to your crown chakra and visualize a golden orb spinning gently above it. When ready, after your initial assessment, bring this orb down the vertical power current and into the center of the chakra that you know needs clearing.

Gently open this chakra (both the front and the back). Set the intention that this golden light energy instantly transmute all lower vibrational energies.

Use your inhale to strengthen the golden energy orb. As you exhale, allow golden energy to gently "push" or pulse through the chakra, moving from the inside out (from the back of the chakra, connected to the vertical power current, outward to the open front "face" of the chakra). Pulsing energy through the chakra instantly clears and transmutes those lower energies.

When complete, dilate back your chakra to a normal level and allow the golden orb to drop down the vertical power current to create a grounding connection. Then seal your aura and open your eyes.

You can do this exercise with one chakra at a time, or you can work through all of your seven main chakras, moving from top to bottom. Depending on the energy in each chakra, it may take as little as a minute to clear one—or possibly an entire session focusing on just one chakra. Take your time and practice. You can use this method daily or as often throughout the day as you need.

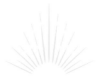

Exercise: Chakra Clearing and Balancing Using Your Hands from the Outside In

With this method, we will be directing channeled healing energy into the chakras in order to help ground the energy down, out, and away from your system. This method is great to use if you feel you can work more easily with your hands than through visualization. It can also be useful for helping to release some of the bigger or denser blocks in the chakras.

Set up your space and find a comfortable seated posture. Set your intention to clear, heal, and balance your chakras.

Take a moment to gently close your eyes and meditate. Bring in your healing light column or white light bubble (page 94 and 96).

Take a moment to establish your grounding connection. This is *very important* for this exercise because that is how the denser energy can leave your system. Once established, expand your grounding cord to the width of your body and open your foot chakras to 100 percent.

Now, rub your palms together vigorously to activate your palm chakras, then let your hands relax.

Bring your awareness to your crown chakra, and gently let it open. Visualize a consistent stream of golden energy running down from your stellar chakra, through your vertical power current into your crown, then flowing through the pathways into your hand chakras.

Use your breathing to inhale the light and then exhale, pulsing it out of your hands. When your hands feel warm or tingle, place your palms facing each other one to two inches apart and oscillate the hands closer and further (about a centimeter of movement). See if you can actively feel the energy "pushing back" between your palms. It should feel similar to pushing together two magnets of the same charge.

Now set the intention that you will be clearing the lower vibrations in your chakras, using your hands and allowing these old energies to flow down your grounding cord into the core of the Earth for transmutation.

When ready, after your initial assessment, move your hands two to four inches in front of the particular chakra that you know needs clearing. From here, gently dilate open this chakra and use your breathing to send golden light into the open chakra.

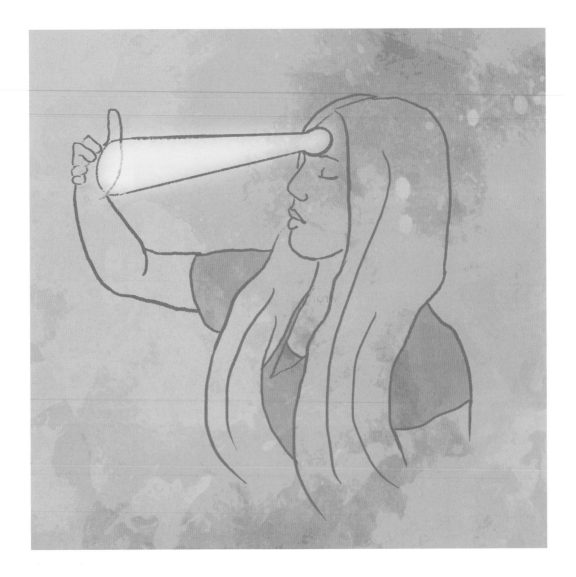

As you inhale, you pull in more light through the crown into your hands, and as you exhale, you gently pulse the energy into the open chakra. Visualize all blocks or static energy being "flushed" directly down the vertical power current (past your root chakra, past the earth star chakra, down your grounding cord), moving directly into the core of the Earth. Only the new healthy golden energy now remains in its place.

Do this breathing for a few rounds until you feel there is no longer any discordant energy in the chakra.

When complete, dilate your chakra back to a normal level, regulate your crown chakra back to a normal dilation, and then seal your aura and open your eyes.

After you've tried both methods, journal about them and reflect on your experience. Was there one method you preferred over the other? What was it like for you to work with your hands? What did you "feel" or sense during your session?

———————

This method works from the outside, inward, where we pulse energy into the front of the open chakra to the back, where it connects in to the vertical power current. You can do this with one chakra at a time per session or you can do your entire system. When working with this outside-in approach, I recommend starting from the root upward, as its best to clear the blocks in the lower chakras first so the energy can properly flow down the vertical power current and ground off into the Earth.

There is no "right" or "wrong" way to do this practice. One method is not superior to the other; they are just different approaches that work in different ways. The first method is the best way to go if you'd like to focus more on bringing the energy upward and for things like enlightenment or a kundalini awakening. (Kundalini awakening is where the life force energy is sitting dormant at the base of the spine, moves upward through the vertical power current, passing through each open and unblocked chakra, to eventually reach through the crown chakra where divine union with the Universe or Oneness/ Nirvana occurs.) Use the second method if you'd like to focus more on grounding and rooting your energy.

If you're planning on working with all seven chakras in one sitting, give yourself at least forty to sixty minutes of time to complete the process. It may take time to build up to this exercise, which is why we did *so much* preparation and meditation beforehand. With a daily meditation practice, the length of this exercise should feel like a breeze. If you get very sleepy during the session, split up the exercise and start with the upper or the lower chakras first, then end your session and pick up where you left off the next day.

Decoding the Different Sensations in the Palm Chakras

While working with the hands to clear energy, you may experience different sensations in the palm chakras while scanning for blocks or pulsing energy into an area. This is perfectly normal and actually a good sign that your sensitivity level is increasing!

When you're scanning an area and come across a change in temperature, hot or cold, that is a distinct indication of old stagnant energy that needs to be cleared. Tingles or strong pulses in your hand or a feeling of static electricity is also an indicator that you've found some energy that needs to be cleared. Continue sending the energy into that area until these sensations subside.

Here's a little tip to help clear your hands after working with some heavier energies: When you're done with your session, wash your hands with cold water. Set the intention that the water is now cleansing the old energy from your hands as it flushes down the drain.

Clearing and Healing the Aura

The aura is not just one bubble around you. It is multilayered and multifaceted. Each individual layer has its own unique qualities and properties. When working in the aura, you can either work on one layer at a time or you can do the whole aura. You may find differences in each layer: some may feel clean and clear; others may need a lot of clearing, healing, or repair.

It's usually easier to feel and sense the layers closest to the body, as they are more dense. The further outward we move from the body, the more subtle the aura becomes. This is because each layer moves from the lowest, slowest vibration closest to the body (first layer), outward to the highest, fastest vibrations furthest away from the body (seventh layer).

We can only feel or sense up to the dimensional level, or layer of the aura, that *we can hold ourselves*. For example, if we are primarily holding a third dimensional consciousness, then we'll be able only to sense and feel up to the third (dimensional) layer of the aura. This is why we do so much preparation and daily practice to still our mind and bring in more light—to raise our frequency, giving us more available levels to work with in these exercises.

Each auric layer holds its own energy and lessons and by reviewing the different meanings in chapter 2, you'll be able to understand what is happening in your own personal plasmic energy field when you realize which layers you're consistently working on healing. You can work visually with intention and energy from the inside out, or work with your hands, pulsing energy into the aura to clear, boost, or heal the aura.

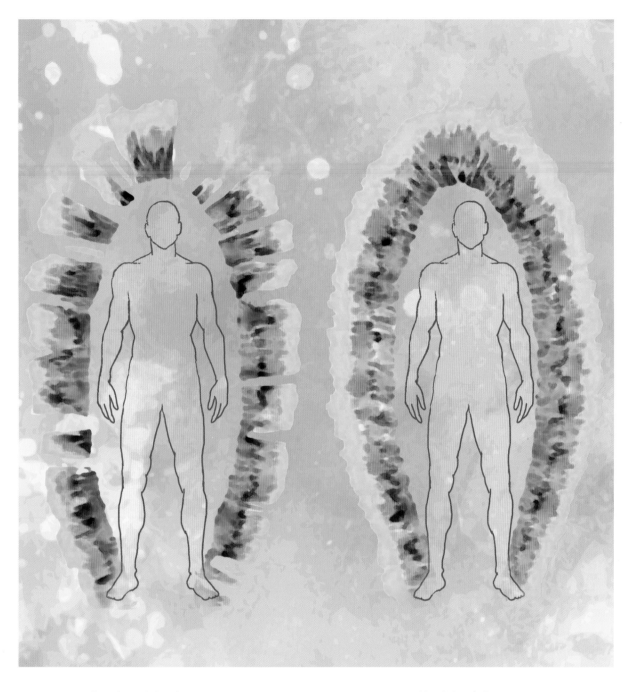

Depleted, broken aura   Healthy, full aura

Exercise: Clear and Strengthen Each Layer

Healing and strengthening our auric field is essential when it comes to having strong energetic protection and boundaries in our daily life. In this exercise, we briefly move through each layer to intentionally boost and create more strength in our fields.

Set up your space and find a comfortable seated posture. Set your intention to clear, heal, and boost your auric field.

Take a moment to gently close your eyes and meditate. Bring in your healing light column or white light bubble (page 94 or 96) before beginning.

Now, bring your awareness to your stellar chakra and visualize a stream of golden light coating the body. This golden light is working on the first layer of the aura, filling up any areas of depletion and instantly transmuting any disruptions or discordant energy. Allow this light to rain down from the stellar chakra, over the head, down the body, and under the feet.

Once you feel this process is complete, then move onto the second layer of the aura, about two inches further away from the body, repeating this same process. You can imagine a golden layer of translucent light coating and filling up each layer as you go. This light will remain here for the next day, gently strengthening your field as it dissolves into each layer.

Continue this exercise with each layer, finishing at the seventh. When complete, ground your energy back in the present time and gently open your eyes.

Journal about your experience, including which layers you could see, feel, or sense during your session. Did you notice anything about one layer over the other? What experiences occurred for you while cleaning your energy?

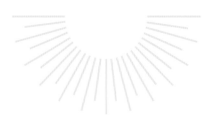

Exercise: Using Your Hands to Charge Your Aura

This exercise is a wonderful alternative for those who prefer working with their hands or have a much easier time "sensing" energy than "seeing" energy. We also have the ability to bring through stronger amounts of energy directly to particular areas of the aura when working with the laser-like quality of our palm chakras.

Set up your space and find a comfortable seated posture. Set your intention to clear, heal, and boost your auric field.

Take a moment to gently close your eyes and meditate. Bring in your healing light column or white light bubble (page 94 or 96) before beginning.

Rub your hands together to activate your palm chakras, and breathe in golden light from your crown down into your hands. Use your exhales to pulse light through the palm chakras. When ready, sense the differences in your auric field with your hands. Can you feel the border of each layer pressing against one another? Can you feel or sense certain areas of depletion (where it feels like there's energy missing) or any hot or cold or prickly spots? Work here.

Send beautiful golden light into this area until you feel the temperature or condition stabilize, then search for the next layers. This approach is more intuitive, as you are "feeling" your way through the aura to heal it.

Continue this exercise throughout the aura, including the back and under your feet and above your head. If you cannot reach an area, *intend* to beam or send the golden light directly to that area instead. Remember, intention is everything and energy can move instantly across time and space (and yes, through matter) when working quantumly.

When you feel this process is complete, ground your energy back into the present time and gently open your eyes.

Journal about your experience, including which layer borders you could feel or sense during your session. What experiences, emotions, or thoughts came up for you while cleaning your energy? Usually this is what was being cleared.

You can work with these exercises as often as you choose. The first approach can take you ten to twenty minutes. The second approach can take longer, but both are very effective. Remember, a healthy, full aura is your best form of energetic protection, so balance the work you've been doing on your chakras along with continuously keeping your aura strong, clear, and bright.

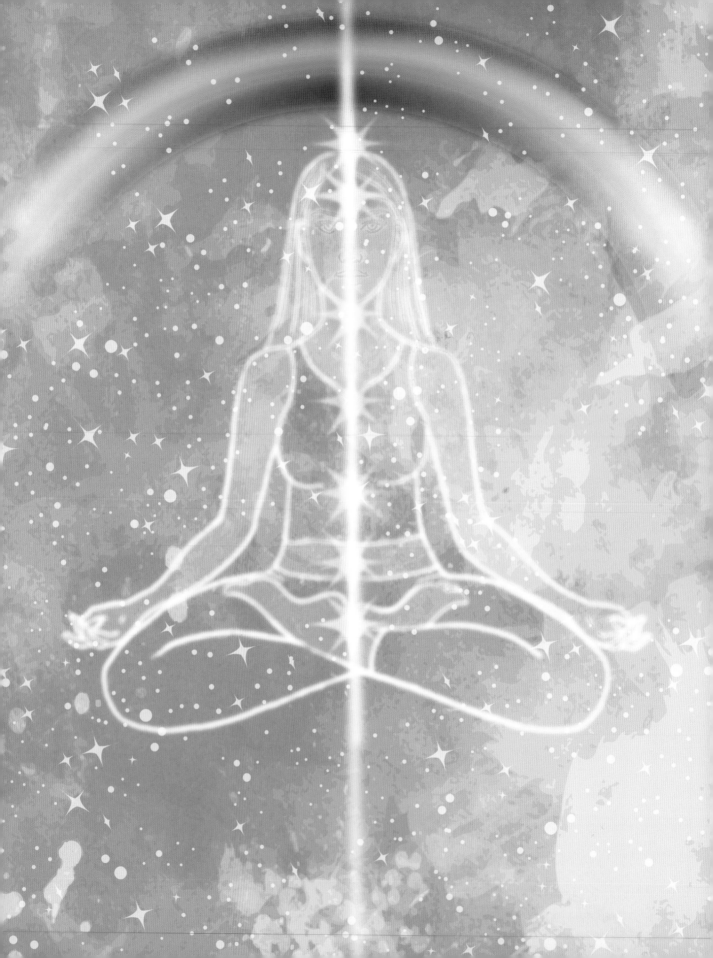

9

Advanced Energy Healing Practices

●

Congratulations on moving into the advanced exercises section. These practices require a higher level of intuitive awareness. You'll also need greater sensitivity to energy, using one or any combination of these gifts: sensitivity in your hands, third eye vision, sentience, extrasensory hearing and/or a knowing, or a strong ability to clearly download and receive the information needed.

It's important to feel a solid ability to create a stable, protective light field around you, ground, and use your ascension column, chakras, and hands to sense and send energy. If that still feels challenging, then continue practicing the exercises in the previous chapter, along with longer periods of meditation, for the next few weeks to clear and boost your energy field before moving forward.

For each exercise that follows, you'll set up your space, physically and energetically, then ground and take a few deep breaths to move into a place of stillness. Moving forward, when you read "take a moment to set yourself up," this is what that entails. From there, we will set individual intentions and then begin each exercise.

Lightbody and DNA Activations

We have worked with the individual aspects of the energy body bit by bit to clear and strengthen our individual chakras and boost our overall field. Now, we will be connecting with the energy of our Soul, or the truest, highest aspect of who we are. Our Soul is multidimensional and exists in many places at once. Our Soul energy can reside in different dimensions, spaces, and realities, having different levels of awareness and experiences all at once. The Soul is the purest level of the Creator or God that dwells within our physical experience and it is eternal.

What is the difference between the spirit and the Soul? The spirt is the energy that surrounds and encases the Soul and can move with it during its many incarnations; it carries the energetic information of the experiences throughout all time and is what fills our physical body and auric field. The Soul itself is a high-vibrational, pure, and individualized fractal of the creative Source of all things. It is the purest part of us, our "spark of God" within, that connects us back to where we all originally came from, and acts as an infinite Source or spring of beautiful, divine energy we can tap into at any time.

The entire practice of the eight-limbed path of yoga, and so many other Eastern practices and religions, is the science (or methodology) of self-realization, or to know oneself. Here we're speaking of the Self with a capital S, meaning the Soul within, not the lower egoic personality self, or the lower or smaller self. To know the Self is to know God, and thus to know all of creation, since we are all a fractalized portion of that cosmic infinite energy within.

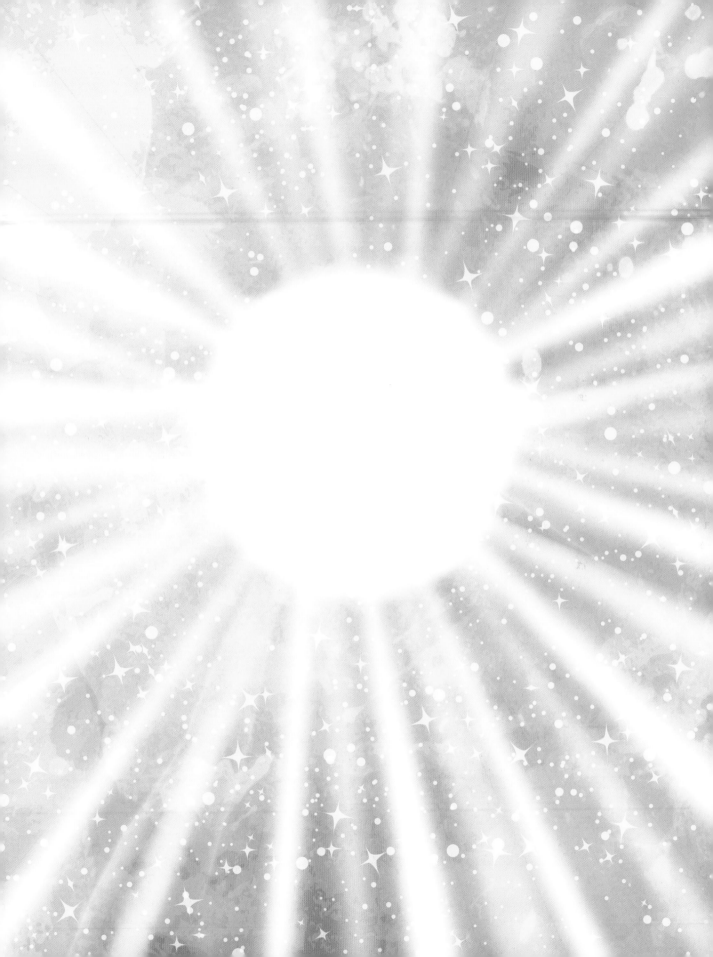

Each time we consciously connect with the high-vibrational energy of our Soul (most easily done when meditating in silence), we can shine and hold more of its light in our physical body. To fully merge with the energy of our Soul and bring its full light potential into our conscious physical experience and awareness is en-lighten-ment. This takes time, dedication, and practice and for many, lifetimes of effort to achieve.

Initially, it's helpful to become familiar with your own Soul's frequency and gently bring in more and more light over time. As you've read, the Soul is multidimensional and exists in many places at once. We can access the energy of our Soul in many ways, usually the most easily through our sacred heart, our soul star chakra, and through activating our divine, etheric (meaning nonphysical) higher dimensional strands of DNA.

What Are Light Codes?

When connecting with our Soul energy or any higher vibrational source of light energy—our sun, the grand central sun (or Source), our higher selves, our spirit guides, or the Akashic Records—we receive, or download, light codes. This intelligent light information comes in larger quantities all at once, similar to receiving a zip file that contains many folders of information and files within.

When these downloads of light codes occur, we often hear a subtle tone in one ear only, that usually lasts only around ten to fifteen seconds, or our eyes may move rapidly, similar to when in REM sleep. Often, these downloads occur unconsciously or spontaneously every night as we're sleeping. This is why so often we wake up with a new idea, an answer to our problem, or an understanding that we did not have before.

When connecting with the energy of our Soul, it is very common to receive these downloads as a by-product of this connection. When this occurs, place your hands over your heart and offer gratitude for the experience that is occurring, as it is a blessing.

Also note that these light code downloads take time to unpack, as they are "coded" with large amounts of subtle, spiritual information. The best way to "decode" them is to let them open and unfold at their own pace, as each bit of intelligent information will unlock at the right time, according to your own personal consciousness level at the moment. Pushing or trying to force the information forward won't help reveal it any faster. Rest and relax—or meditate—and give thanks for your newfound connection with higher levels of light intelligence.

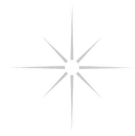

Exercise: Bringing in More of Your Personal Soul Energy with the Soul Star Chakra

In the following exercise, we will be intentionally connecting with the energy of our Soul to bring more of our own higher light into the physical body. So, take a moment to set yourself up physically and energetically, and then ground and center yourself before beginning. This exercise will take five to ten minutes.

Once grounded and centered, set the intention to lovingly connect with and bring the energy and light of your own Soul into your physical body. If you choose, you may call in your guides, higher self, or archangels Michael or Metatron for additional protection. Only do this if it resonates with you.

Then take a few moments to bring your conscious awareness to your heart chakra. You can put your hands on your heart and take a few moments to breathe here. When ready, gently release your hands onto your lap.

Visualize a bright golden light shining at the center of your heart chakra: this represents your conscious awareness. Now visualize this golden light slowly moving up the vertical power current to the higher heart charka, then the throat chakra, past the third eye, and to the crown; take a breath here.

From here, using your intention, visualize this golden light of your awareness slowly traveling up the vertical power current to about two feet above the crown chakra, then into your soul star chakra. You may see this chakra as a beautiful gemlike magenta or white-golden light, or feel the energy of this chakra as high-vibrational warm, loving energy. You may hear a tone or simply get a knowing that your awareness is "in" your soul star chakra.

Notice what you're feeling. What are you experiencing in this moment? What does your personal Soul frequency look, sound, and feel like to you? Trust the information you receive.

Take a few deep breaths for about a minute or two (or as long as you can handle without getting sleepy) with the intention of letting beautiful shimmering light codes flow down from your soul star chakra into your crown, like a glittering column of rain.

When you're ready, slowly travel the tiny golden light of your awareness back down the vertical power current into the crown chakra and take a breath, then down into the third eye chakra and do the same, moving down each chakra until you reach the heart, taking a full breath in and out at each one.

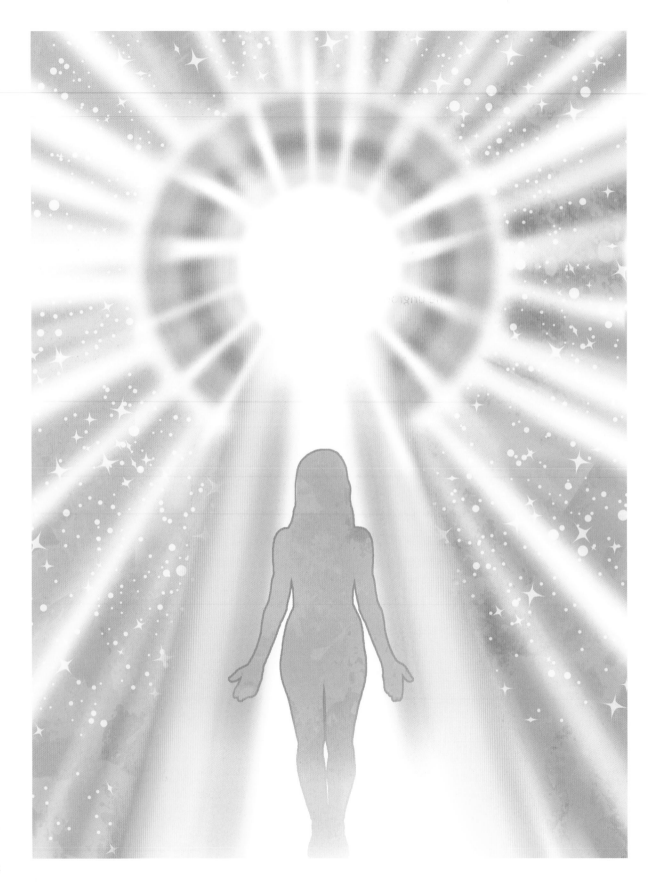

Breathe here for a moment and notice how your energy feels now. Sometimes when we connect with such a high frequency it can feel like we're humming or vibrating with positive energy. Meditate here for as long as you'd like.

When ready, reground yourself by energetically connecting back into the Earth, moving yourself back into the present time. Refortify the outer edge of your aura, and then slowly open your eyes. Give thanks for the connection and then journal what you experienced.

This is a powerful and simple exercise that will gradually allow you to bring more and more of your Soul's light into the body. You can do this daily at the beginning of your meditations for the first few minutes or after you have properly set up your space and energy and grounded.

It is easy to become ungrounded and to want to stay up in these higher vibrational spaces after an exercise like this. It is not safe physically or energetically to have your awareness outside of your body after finishing these exercises, so it is very important to make sure that you energetically reground yourself at the end of each exercise—and to make sure you are fully back in your body and aware before moving on with your day.

Signs That You Are Not Fully Grounded

Some signs you are *not* in your body may include:

- You feel "spacy," light-headed, or "up in the clouds."
- You are forgetful or clumsy (e.g., bumping into things, having trouble speaking or typing properly).
- You may have an overall feeling of slight dizziness or may feel "out of it" (because you *literally* are).

Do not drive or operate machinery until you are fully grounded back into your body in the present time. If you're having trouble grounding back in properly, refer to page 105 for alternative, easy ways to ground. This is a beautiful, sacred experience that in time will strengthen and deepen the connection with your Soul.

Psychic Surgery and Removing Energy Blocks

Once you've cleared the energy centers and aura, and have brought in more and more high-vibrational light, you may notice certain areas in or around the body or in the energy field where you feel slight pressure, a change in temperature, or something feels "off." These are the deeper-seated energetic blocks that have most likely been there for a long time (think early childhood or possibly later). You'll know you have a deeper energy block if you find that over the course of several exercises you notice a sensation or see the same image in the same part of the body or aura over and over.

In this chapter, you'll learn to identify the block and make sure you're willing to release it. Gently release the block through your set chosen energetic technique and dispose of the energy properly. And finally, you'll charge or fill up the area that has been worked on with high-vibrational light.

Energy healing happens in layers and that is why we left clearing the deeper-seated energetic traumas and blocks for the advanced section. It is very important that you have been slowly clearing your energy and bringing in more and more light, so you won't overwhelm the system. If you clear everything too quickly, you may end up missing layers altogether.

Energetic blocks typically come from old, stuck experiences, belief systems, traumas, memories, or unexpressed or sustained lower emotional energies held in the body instead of being released. Energetic blocks can be found anywhere in the physical body, organs, and tissues. They can also be found in the chakras, channels, meridians, or anywhere in the auric field.

These blocks do what they say—they literally "block" the proper flow of energy from moving throughout the body. When this happens over time, it usually translates as physical pain in that region, a weakness in that area, psychological issues, or even a serious health issue or disease in the body.

Identifying the Block

Most of the time these blocks are formed and maintained unconsciously, until very high-vibrational light is introduced, which comes in and illuminates the contrast of energies. As we raise our frequency, the older, toxic, and disharmonious energies we have carried are no longer a resonant match for our higher vibration.

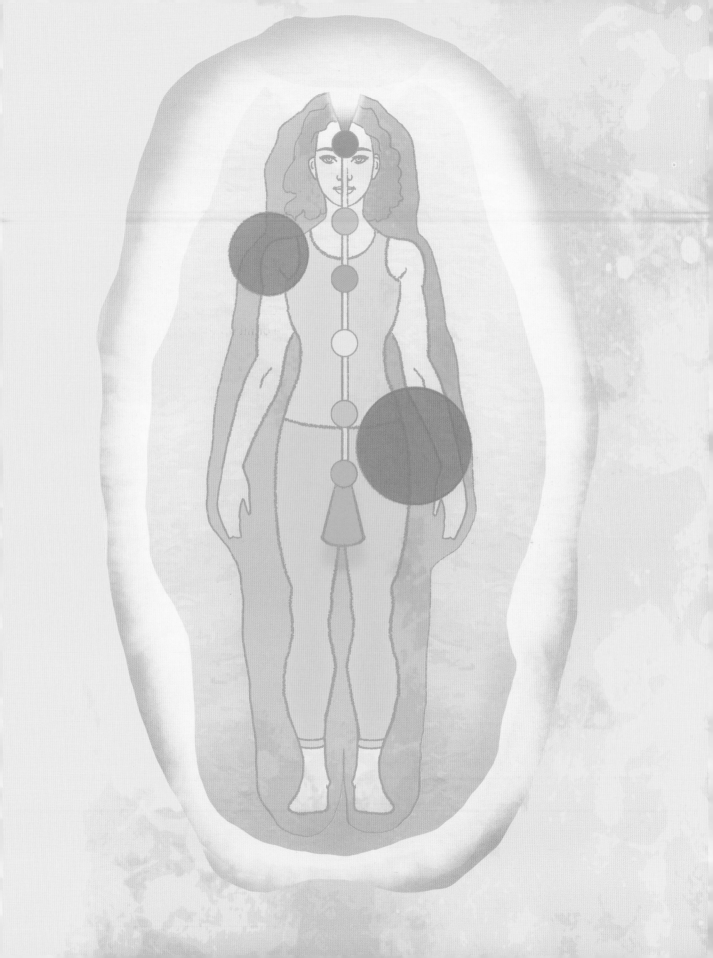

This is why when we start working on our energy and "turning the light on," so to speak, it can feel like all of a sudden we have so much to do right away. But that's not how energy healing works in most cases (except for miraculous healing, like instant spontaneous remission). It's very important to pace yourself along the way. These things were already there, and just like a massage, you want to slowly warm up and gently release the tension in the superficial layers of the muscles first, before breaking up the deeper knots or long-standing patterns in the fascia and tissues—doing this in reverse would just be painful.

In addition to noticing, feeling, or seeing where a block may be located during your previous sessions, or through dowsing with your pendulum, you can set the intention to identify the blocks in your system before you begin. An energetic block can look and feel like anything, depending on its origin. For some people, it can literally feel like a concrete block; for others, it's like a toy block if it's from childhood. It can even look like an engagement ring if it came from a divorce or a dagger if that person felt "stabbed in the back" by another. It's okay if you can't discern the exact size or shape or color of the block. What is important is that you identify and discern that the energy is not flowing properly in the location and that it "feels" or looks off to you.

How to Preform Psychic Surgery

There are a few steps to follow when working on clearing these deep-seated blocks. The block may be different each time, but the methods to clearing and healing it will typically be the same. This method is derived in part from the Reiki master technique.

1. **Identify exactly what it is you're looking to release.**

   You may go into meditation and ask your higher self these questions: Where is the block located? What does it look like? Where did it originate (age, time period, what happened)? Is there any additional information you need to know about it to release it? Get as detailed as you need to.

2. **Ask yourself: Am I willing and ready to release this block?**

   This may entail forgiving someone from your past or forgiving yourself, or it may involve having to shift your belief systems around a particular situation that may have been the cause. It is very important to have the willingness to release the block; otherwise, practicing any of the below exercises will not work. If you discover it's something that you're not willing to release yet, that's all right too. Give it time, and do the inner work to see how it's serving you to keep it. Then and only then, move forward when ready.

3. **Begin to gently and slowly remove the energetic block from the system using one technique from below (choose intuitively).**

   With practice, you'll find the methods that work best for you depending on the different blocks you encounter. Once you have removed the block, dispose of the energy properly, so it doesn't return or remain in your space where you are clearing it.

4. **Refill or "charge" the areas with high-vibrational light after you have cleared them.**

   Whatever area has been worked on will now be open or "vacant," since the block previously there has now been removed. The Universe hates a vacuum. Where there is empty space, the Universe will immediately try to fill that void. So, it's important to refill or "charge" these areas with high-vibrational light. If you don't, you are leaving an opening in your energy field where literally anything could enter. When you are "charging up" the area, keep sending energy until you feel that area has been completely filled. The time process for this may vary depending on the depth and size of the block that was released.

Sometimes, when working with deeply rooted blocks, you may find you have to work in layers in one sitting to fully remove the entire block. Psychic surgery is a skill and can be used for energies beyond just blocks in the system, but it takes a very practiced and experienced practitioner to see and release the more deeply embedded external energies from within the different layers of the aura or physical tissues. Practicing these methods will help you develop your skills for releasing these blocks on your own.

Sometimes during a release, you may experience emotions or physical sensations releasing along with the block. It is very common to cry or have older emotions or memories come to the surface (to clear) while releasing the block, even if they do not make linear sense why. It is also common to physically "feel" the work being done on that area of the body or occasionally, even out in the aura.

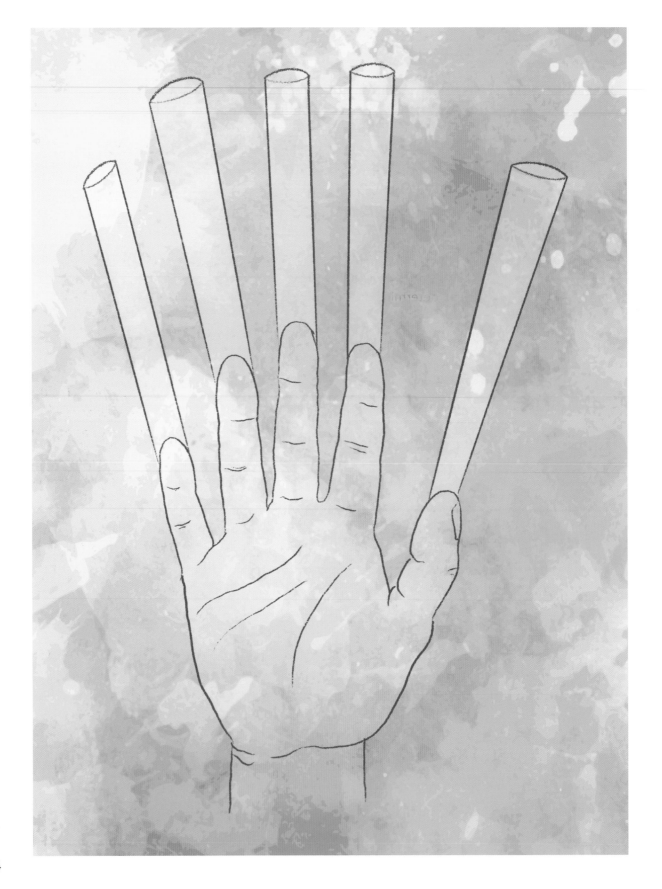

Exercise: Releasing Energy Blocks

As you learn these techniques, start each exercise by setting up your physical and energetic space, finding stillness and grounding, with the option of connecting in with your team, higher self, or the archangels for assistance. Set the intention to be shown, to feel, or to know about any energy blocks that need to be released from your system. Then identify and get clear on what exactly it is you're looking to release. You can go into meditation for this for anywhere from five to thirty to get the information you need. Then, the process of completing the three steps to release the energy block can take thirty minutes to an hour, depending on the block.

Part 1: Different Techniques for Releasing Blocks with Energy

Once you are set up, make sure you have identified your block, gained the information needed on it, and determined that you are ready to release it at this time.

Take a moment to activate your palm chakras by gently rubbing them together. Rest your palms face up on your lap. Bring high-vibrational golden light in through your crown and channel it out from your palm chakras.

Golden Gloves. Your first option for psychic surgery is to use this golden light to "build" or create golden gloves all around your hands, with a thick layer of golden energy around each finger, down to your wrists. Once they are "on," you can use your hands to go into the area to release the block from your energy field.

This technique usually works best when the block is closer to the surface of the body, is in the aura, or is bigger or bulkier.

Etheric Fingers. A second option is to extend your etheric fingers, or energetic fingers, out longer from your hands. You can do this by simply visualizing the golden light moving from your palms and out from your fingers, or you can gently "pull" each etheric energy finger out from the top of the finger pad (they are usually six to twelve inches long). Either way, it will look and feel like you have finger extensions or the longest nails ever. Picture these etheric fingers operating like mini tongs to extract the block.

Use this technique if the block is deeper in the body, smaller or more refined, or looks like something that you don't want to touch.

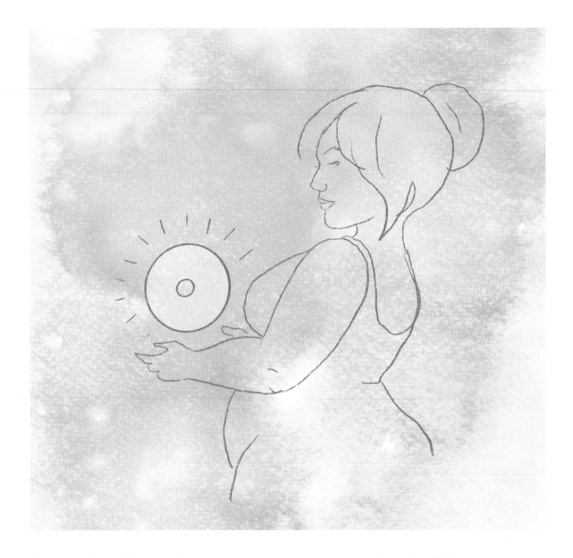

Golden Bubble. Your third option is to create a hollow golden orb of light using your hands. We'll be calling this a golden bubble. Using your palm chakras and your breathing, rub your hands together for a bit and then keep them still and separate them so they are just barely touching. Concentrate on this area and picture a tiny golden light bubble between your palms. As you breathe in, bring golden light in and down into your palm chakras. As you exhale, gently expand your hands wider, slowly creating or "stretching" your bubble out wider.

Once your bubble is a little bit bigger than the size of your block, and holding it like a beach ball, gently and slowly surround the block with this golden bubble. You may see or feel this bubble. Initially, you may have to visualize it and trust it is working until your sensitivities develop. From here, slowly lift or "sweep" the block now contained within your bubble up and away from the body or auric field.

This method is best used for blocks in the chakras or bigger blocks in the energy field that are deeply lodged in the body, but can be used for blocks of any size.

Part 2: Properly Disposing of the Negative Energy

Once the block is out of your body or system, beam light onto it to slowly dissolve it. There are a few options for how to do this.

Breath-Centered Method. Use your breathing to dissolve the energy. Inhale and bring in golden light from your crown. Exhale, sending the light out from your palms onto the older energy block. With a few breaths (depending on the size of the block), it will slowly dissolve.

Working with the Elements. Another option is to work with the elements, such as the energy of fire, and visualize the block being burned into ash from the fire. Once complete, energetically put your fire out.

The Violet Flame. You can work with violet energy to dispose of the energy. Picture surrounding the block within a violet flame of energy or within a large orb of vibrant violet light to dissolve it. You can also beam the violet energy all around and into the block until it dissolves completely.

Releasing to the Light. You may also lift the block high, up toward the sky, with the intention of releasing the block up into the light. You can also ask your spirit guides, higher self, or the angels to take this block from you and assist with its clearing.

The method you use may depend on the block. Usually, the smaller blocks are easy to dissolve with light. The more challenging blocks may need the violet flame or the assistance of an angel to help you properly dispose of the energy.

Signs You Have Released a Block

- A deep sigh of relief

- Feeling a "weight" coming off of you

- Energetically or physically feeling "lighter," happier, or more peaceful

Part 3: Charging the Area with Light

When you've finished dissolving or disposing of the block, return to the area that has been worked on. Send healing golden energy back into that region. Use your breathing to channel in and send out the golden light from your hands. Take as much time as you need to do this until the area feels "full" and complete. If you felt tenderness around the physical region or had a lot of emotions release from the experience, you can also bring in beautiful, vibrant emerald light, which holds the energy of healing.

You may notice, after charging for a bit, that there are additional areas that come up to be released and cleared. If so, repeat the above exercises, then follow up with charging the area again.

Once the charging is complete, you can "remove" or dissolve your golden gloves or retract your etheric fingers, then reground your energy and seal your auric field.

When your session is complete, drink a glass of water to assist with the grounding and detoxification process. You can also wash your hands with the intention of clearing any old energy that may have gotten through.

At the end of the experience, give thanks for your ability to release the old and bring in the new. Take notes on anything you may have experienced or felt during or after the exercise.

Congratulations on completing your first round of psychic surgery! Practice each of the three techniques used to release the blocks to see what works best for you. Then separately try the different techniques for disposing of the blocks individually to see what works best. These techniques aren't "one size fits all." Even if you become used to a certain technique or prefer one over the other, it will be helpful for you to be proficient in all of them, so you can use them for the different blocks and different circumstances that arise.

Psychic surgery is a skill. The more you practice, the better you will become at it and the easier it will be to go through the steps. Do pace yourself when it comes to the deeper clearings, and give yourself time between sessions to rest and integrate the energetic changes into the physical body. For lighter sessions, this can be one to three days; for deeper sessions, this can be four to eight weeks. You can use your pendulum to dowse and find out the integration time, or ask and intuitively receive the information in your meditation.

Removing Energy Cords

Energy cords are energetic tubes or tunnels of light energy between two parties where energy, thoughts, and emotions are exchanged at an instantaneous speed. Some cords can be useful and helpful in relationships, such as that between a mother and her newborn or child, or a pet parent with their pet. But having energy cords can be very draining and toxic to the energetic system. Picture energy cords like having a direct landline or cable connecting you to the other party, nonstop, where the phone is open all the time—it's exhausting and can be downright uncomfortable. We don't need to be leaking our energy outward or receiving incoming energy from external sources at all times of day.

Our last exercise of the book is to develop skills for releasing energetic cords. Energy cords are complex, and removing them is not as simple as karate chopping them or pulling them out. There is an in-depth process to releasing cords, and some even involving releasing long-standing energy contracts from the past. Releasing energy cords can change someone's life for the better and help them move forward from relationships, places, jobs, or scenarios in their life that are "tying them down" or where codependency occurs.

We can form energy cords to other people, places, and things, and even different times or memories in our lives. Cords usually form due to an intense emotional exchange of energy between two parties. This can be as simple as a quick, heated exchange with a person that bumps into you on the street. Or it might be a stored traumatic memory from a past event. It could be a best friend you have to share every last detail with, or previous romantic partners you were intimate with. (Let me be clear: you most definitely will have formed a cord with anyone that you have ever been sexually intimate with.)

Cords can form in an instant and will remain there unless the person has consciously released it or the relationship. Sometimes this decision alone can work to release cords. Most of the time, the deeply embedded or long-standing cords need to be consciously energetically released.

The thing about cording is that on a higher level, it is always a mutual decision. The only things that can enter our fields are things we allow to enter for many reasons. Some of these are physical, potentially due to our defenses being down due to stress, sadness, or lack of sleep. Others are subconscious and energetic, meaning that even though you say you are over the relationship and never want to see them again, deep down subconsciously you do, and so the cord remains or keeps returning. If there's a cord, it's there for a reason, and it is usually serving both parties in some capacity until it's not anymore.

Different Levels and Types of Cords

Different types of energy cords can occur between two parties. The first is the most basic energy cord, which was described above. It usually extends from one party to the other and plugs in on both sides. These cords can be long inside the body or short and easy to remove; it all correlates with the intensity and length of the energy exchange at hand. Then there are much smaller energy cords, sometimes called "feelers" or "streamers," that reach out like little antennas into someone else's personal space when they are not necessarily welcome. This usually occurs unconsciously, and we usually see these in small groups or bundles. The last type of energy cord is called a hook, because it usually has an energetic form of a fishhook, or multiple fishhooks, at one end. Hooks usually occur out of desperation, when one party feels desperate to keep the other party on the line and attached to them; they are usually (subconsciously) accepted by the other party because they are too fearful to break the connection and walk away.

Signs You Have an Energy Cord

- You can't stop thinking of the person or situation.

- You get thoughts that aren't yours.

- You have a negative or slightly painful feeling in a particular chakra or area of the body when thinking of the person or situation.

- You suddenly feel emotions that aren't yours.

- You think of them and they immediately reach out or vice versa.

- You just don't feel like "yourself."

- You feel like you can't move forward in life because something is holding you back (and it most definitely is).

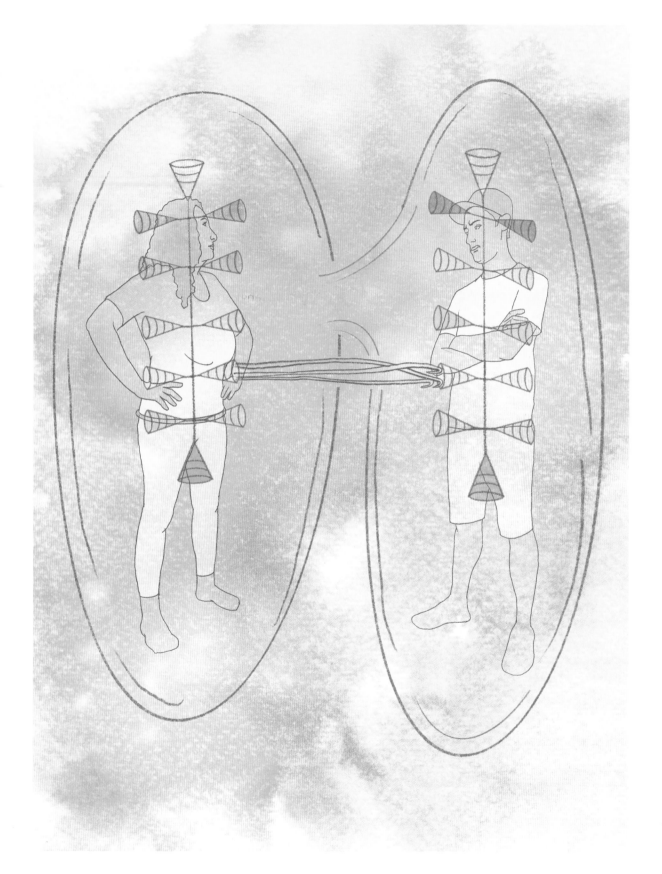

It's always important to remember that we do have conscious control over our energy field and who or what we let in, as opposed to believing we are the victims of these external energies that have come our way. Even with hooks, there is almost always an (unconscious) energetic agreement made on a higher plane by the spirits of the parties involved to allow this energetic exchange. These can be the trickiest to release, as the conventional method of pulling or cutting cords won't work on releasing these denser stuck energies.

It takes discernment, clarity, and honesty with oneself to handle energy cords. You need to fully understand the situation at hand to clearly see or intuit and identify the cord, its cause, and the connection to the other party to release the cord permanently. If you discover a cord that you'd like to keep instead of releasing it, you can simply run light through it to clear it. (I don't recommend this, unless it's with a mother and young child, as it can create energetic interference and codependence.) That said, if you're setting the proper intentions to be shown cords that need to be released, then trust what you're seeing is ready to go—it wouldn't be revealed to you otherwise.

Most of the time when working in sessions, you usually need to know who or what the cord is attached to, and why, to begin releasing it. This isn't always the case, as I have found exceptions to this when people are ready to move forward in their life by finally releasing their past and allow everything that is no longer serving their highest good to go. Occasionally, just setting powerful intentions to release all cording, made purely from the heart, can be enough to help it release. This is the exception, as some of the deeper, long-standing cords need an active release through these techniques.

Exercise: Safely Remove Energy Cords

To begin releasing a cord, set up your space physically and energetically. Then ground yourself, and go into meditation for a few moments.

Set the intention to see, feel, or know about any cords that are no longer serving your highest good. Then set the intention to release all lower energy cords from your system in this session.

When ready, activate your palm chakras and, using your breathing, fill your hands with golden light. Intend to create golden gloves that surround your hands before beginning this work.

Now identify the cord and its location in the body and intuitively retrieve information on it by asking questions. Where is it in the body? Why is it there? Who or what is on the other side? How long has it been here? How has it been serving you?

See or feel the cord using either your clairvoyance or clairsentience. An easy way to do this is to have your palms facing each other a few inches apart, then to detect the cord, raise one palm higher than the other, and try to cross the midline between your hands. If there is a cord present, it will feel like you're pressing up against something and your hands won't cross. If there is no cord there, they will easily intersect.

See if you can actively see or feel its shape, size, length, and quality. Some cords will feel hot and sticky; others can feel and look spiky or prickly (these are not the good kind). Identifying the qualities of this cord is advanced work because it requires a high skill and sensitivity level to do this. Without being able to interpret this, let alone find the cord, it will be very challenging to properly release it.

Now discern whether this is a mini "feeler," a solid energy cord, or a hook. You can tell by the ease of its release. If you gently tug on it or run your hand down it and it comes right out, then it is typically a feeler. If it's a true energy cord, it may give slightly when you tug on it, but there will be more "rope" or cord to release from where it's plugged into. If it's an energetic hook, then when you gently tug on it, it will barely budge and you may feel the area where the hook is located being pulled on. You may also clairvoyantly see the energetic hook inside the body.

Once you've discerned what type of cord it is, then you can release it. Feelers release easily with a simple tug or a gentle, intentional slow chop in front of them. After this has been done, send healing golden energy to the area where the feelers previously were.

Traditional energy cords usually require a little more work. If the cord is in an area of the body, then use your hands to hold onto the cord and gently pull it out like you would a rope or cable that has been retracted. Keep gently pulling, one hand at a time, until you feel a sense of release in your body and no longer feel the cord in your hands. You can do the same sensing test, where you pass your hands across one another to see if they pass or if there is still a cord there.

Keep going until it's fully gone. This can take one to twenty minutes depending on the length of the cord. If the energy cord is plugged into a chakra, then use one hand to hold down or stabilize the chakra the whole time, as you are slowly pulling the cord out with the other hand. You can also use dowsing to check and see whether your cord has been released or not. After you've released the cord, send light into the affected area, as there is usually a vacant area where the cord used to be plugged in. Depending on the depth and intensity, you can be charging the area for anywhere from a minute to half an hour if necessary, to make sure the entire area is filled with light.

If there is a hook in the system, it's important to first gently dismantle or remove the hook slowly, piece by piece. This takes strong intentions, clairvoyant vision, or extraordinary clairsentience to do. You may also call upon the archangels or your spirit team to assist you with this process. Take your time, either gently breaking and removing the base pieces of the hook or trying to dissolve them with laser-like precision light, which is usually where using a professionally cut quartz crystal wand can come in handy. Only when you have fully broken it off into smaller pieces or dissolved the hook end of the cord you can begin the same process of gently pulling the rest of the cord out. When you have it removed, clean up or excavate any remaining energies or pieces of the hook that may be left over or embedded. You can use your etheric fingers for this process. Then charge this area with golden light until it's full. You may need to do extra repair, creating small stitches of light with your fingers where the previous intrusion was. Only do this is you are being intuitively guided to do so.

When the charging is complete, you can "remove" or dissolve your golden gloves and retract your etheric fingers, and then reground your energy and seal your auric field.

When your session is complete, you can wash your hands, if you choose, with the intention of clearing any old energy that may have gotten through.

At the end of the experience, give thanks for your ability to release the old external attachments and codependency. And give thanks for the newfound sense of peace and sovereignty in your personal energy field. Take notes on anything you may have seen, experienced, or felt during or after this exercise.

If the Cord Returns

After releasing cords, you should feel lighter and brighter, like you have clarity of thought and mind, and more of your own energy back and intact. When releasing cords, it is common to have the person or party on the other end of the cord notice and occasionally reach out, even if you are no longer in contact. This is because you both are no longer leaking and exchanging energy, or in certain cases one can no longer syphon it off from the other, and they notice this.

The work you do with the energy must be backed up by and followed through with in the physical realm. This means if you released a cord with someone energetically, but then choose to text back and forth or engage in emotional exchanges with them afterward, then your actions are not in integrity with your previous work and the cord will form again because of your true desires, shown through your actions. If you release the cord and then decide to no longer remain in contact with this person, or only have limited or neutral verbal exchanges with the person, then you are acting in integrity with your energy, and the results will stick.

Where a cord with a loved one or family member needed to be released, but you still want to continue your relationship, simply set the intention that your relationship will be of love and independence or interdependence, while respecting the other's autonomy. Just because you release a cord does not always mean that the physical relationship will release too; that is a personal free will choice you get to make with each individual relationship you encounter.

In the deeper cases involving marriages and divorces, victim and abuser, or estranged family members, there tends to be a much stronger karmic component to these exchanges. In these cases, sometimes it is necessary to make a declaration of clearing the old energetic contracts made at a much older time in your spiritual path that are no longer serving your highest good. This tends to be work done more effectively while working in the Akashic Records, but it is possible for you to do this on your own with simple intention.

When you're ready, you can say something like, "I now cancel all lower level contracts with _____ , throughout all times, spaces, dimensions, and realities. You go your way, and I go mine. I forgive you; I love you and I thank you for all of the lessons learned. And so it is."

Saying this—and meaning it—with pure heart intention behind it can be all that you need to do to permanently dissolve a cord that has been there for lifetimes. Everything is energy, and one of the most important ways to work with and steer energy into a proper direction is through the power of setting intentions. Here, setting intentions can set you free.

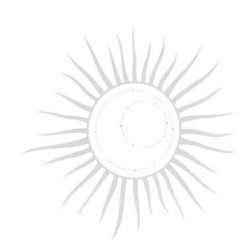

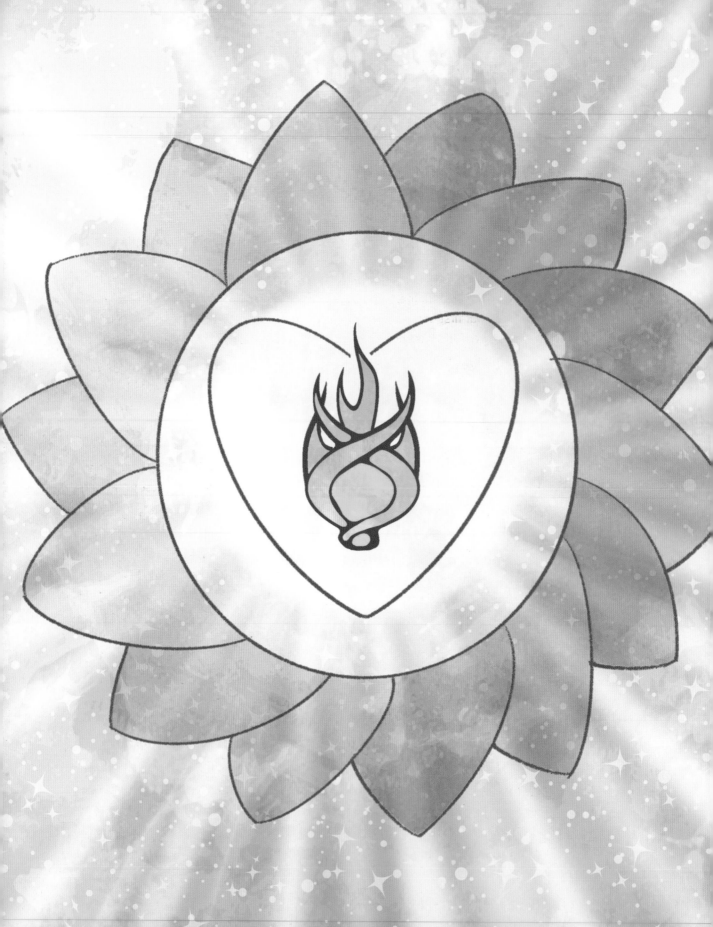

Completing Your Healing Journey

Congratulations! You are well on your way to success on your healing path. This work is not for the faint of heart, and your effort, time, open-mindedness, and courage will help you immensely along the way. You are diving into the depths of your energetic being and becoming aware of your patterns and habits. This is a beautiful time of immense spiritual growth, and I am so, so excited to see you shine your light even brighter.

Through the exercises in this book, you've learned to clear and charge your chakras and aura daily. Stick with this! The more often you clean and clear your energy, the less "work" you'll have to do each time. These energetic hygiene practices will improve the overall quality of your happiness and life. Keep a log of each session, noting how you felt before and after. Reread your first entries: you'll be amazed at how much healing you've done and by how much your life has shifted into one of synchronicity, ease, flow, and grace.

Be extremely proud of yourself for completing the energy healing exercises in this book. And remember: this is just the beginning of your lifelong journey! You have beautiful spiritual gifts available to you in this lifetime, and your daily practices will move you into a new healing direction on your ascension path. Each practice session will peel back layers and develop your intuition. You will learn and understand the true, full picture of who you are inside and release all things that are no longer aligned. Healing your energy can create subtle and powerful positive shifts that will help you reach your highest potential.

Our society is slowly evolving and ascending, and you, my friend, are one of the many wayshowers here to light a path forward in the new golden age that humanity is stepping into. Your work with clearing your energetic field, and building up, strengthening, and shining your inner light, makes more of a difference than you may ever know. There are millions of beautiful light beings cheering for you on the other side that are so happy that another lightworker is discovering their light and moving onto their highest time line. This decision positively affects not only you and your immediate family and loved ones, but also your neighborhood, your community, your country, and, literally, the entire planet.

Thank you for sharing your time and for trusting me as your guide. I am honored to have assisted you on this journey and am looking forward to hearing about all of the spiritual progress and positive energetic shifts that you've made. It is a blessing to us all to have yet another lightworker's beautiful light turned on and shining in the world. The more people who have activated their light, the brighter this world will be.

I'm wishing you much peace, happiness, love, transformation, and success on your wonderful energy healing journey and ascension process to come!

Resources

Energy healing is a broad field, with many different styles and practices that fall underneath it. Here are some of the styles and schools referenced throughout the book. Beneath that are additional resources for those who would like to continue their educational journey and practice with energy healing. Enjoy!

References

Brennan, Barbara Ann. *Hands of Light: A Guide to Healing through the Human Energy Field: A New Paradigm for the Human Being In Health, Relationship, and Disease.* Random House, 1988.

Cooper, Diana, and Tim Whild. *The Archangel Guide to Ascension: Visualizations to Assist Your Journey to the Light.* Hay House, 2015.

Forsyth, Russell, and IEL Institute for the Spiritual Arts: iel-institute.com

McCartney, Francesca. *Body of Health: The New Science of Intuition Medicine for Energy and Balance.* New World Library, 2010.

Rand, William Lee. *Reiki Master Manual: Including Advanced Reiki Training.* Vision Publications, 2003.

Further Reading

Energy Medicine: Balancing Your Body's Energies for Optimal Health, Joy, and Vitality by Donna Eden with David Feinstein, Ph.D.

The Subtle Body: An Encyclopedia of Your Energetic Anatomy by Cyndi Dale

Shaman, Healer, Sage: How to Heal Yourself and Others with the Energy Medicine of the Americas by Alberto Villoldo, Ph.D.

Energy Healing for Animals: A Hands-On Guide for Enhancing the Health, Longevity, and Happiness of Your Pets by Joan Ranquet

Anatomy of the Spirit: The Seven Stages of Power and Healing by Caroline Myss

Creating Sacred Space with Feng Shui: Learn the Art of Space Clearing and Bring New Energy into Your Life by Karen Kingston

Becoming Supernatural: How Common People Are Doing the Uncommon by Dr. Joe Dispenza

The Biology of Belief: Unleashing the Power of Consciousness, Matter & Miracles by Bruce H. Lipton, Ph.D.

The Hidden Messages in Water by Masaru Emoto

You Can Heal Your Life by Louise Hay

Acknowledgments

Thank you, God, the One, the Universe, for providing the opportunity so swiftly and for supporting my calling. I prayed one night to be an instrument of your divine will and was contacted to write this book one week later.

Thank you, Jill, for so synchronistically finding me at just the right time and for all of your continued help and support throughout the process, from conception to the completion of this book. Thank you, Jenna, for your fantastic editing.

Thank you to my beautiful family for your continued support, love, and inspiration along my journey. Deep gratitude to my mother and sister for their unwavering belief in me each time I embarked on a new chapter of my life. Josh, thank you so much for all of your love, support, and encouragement in so many ways, throughout the years, through all our many life changes, and throughout the entire creation, editing, and completion of this book. I love you dearly. To my little but mighty Zeus: Thank you for being my support throughout lifetimes and for warming my heart and helping me smile each and every day.

Gratitude for all of my previous teachers and mentors who assisted me at different points of my personal journey. Thank you to my parents for being my biggest teachers of all. And thank you especially to Mahatmaji for your love and stern teachings while you were here with us and for your continuous support from the other side.

Utmost gratitude to my Higher Self, my team of light, star family, and my spiritual guides residing within the Akashic Records, whose nudge, support, and infinite wisdom inspired me to bring this book into form. Thank you to all of the Archangels and ascended masters who assisted me personally with their love and encouragement throughout the process. I am also thanking myself, for all of the hard work and very late nights spent at the computer in dedication to my mission of raising the collective frequency, which gave me the continuous inspiration for this book. Thank you to all of the beings of light that continuously assist with the transmission, implication, and assimilation of knowledge and positive vibrations coming through the pages of this book. And lastly, I'd like to thank your Higher Self, your spiritual guides, and you, who all conspired together in a beautiful cosmic way to bring you here to finding this book and reading this very page, in this exact moment in "time."

We are all one. Thank you all.

About the Author

Kat Fowler is a light worker, a teacher of spirituality and meditation, an Akashic Records reader and trainer, an advanced Energy Therapist, a Reiki Master Teacher, and host of The Soul Awakening Podcast. Kat has been teaching and mentoring students for over a decade in New York City and internationally. Her life's work is dedicated to raising the frequency of the collective through sharing spiritual practices and healing teachings to help you discover the truest wisdom of your Highest Self, within.

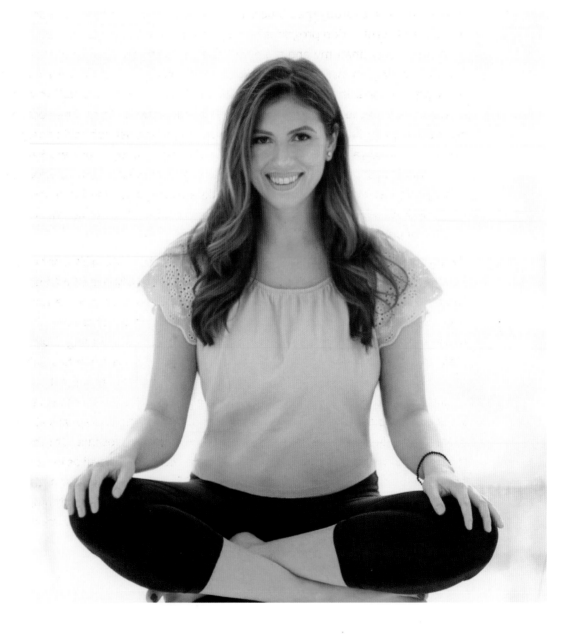

Kat was born into a life of spirituality and meditation: Her parents met in an ashram on their spiritual path. Since birth, Kat was raised as a vegetarian (now she practices veganism) and was connected to yoga philosophy, Eastern spirituality, meditation, and holistic health. She learned meditation through her family's guru at age fourteen. While at college, she specialized in year-long course studies of Yoga Philosophy, Hindu Philosophy, Taoism, the Bhagavad Gita, Buddhist Studies, and Eastern Religions and started practicing yoga at age nineteen. Two years later, Kat began teaching yoga and meditation, and began her journey with energy healing. Soon after, Kat traveled to India to study meditation in depth. Since then, she has taken dozens of training and certification programs; specializing in the Eastern classical elements of yoga, physiology, anatomy, and therapeutics, and additional trainings in Reiki therapy, intuitive healing, animal communication, and advanced energy therapy from several prestigious schools. In addition to her traditional training, Kat has additional studies in Ayurveda, Chinese medicine, psychology, holistic nutrition (including homeopathy), aromatherapy, divination, and crystal therapy. Integrating her upbringing of spirituality and years of dedicated study and teaching, Kat's methodology when working with clients and students in sessions, workshops, and trainings is educational, inspirational, and informative. Her workshops, courses, and talks are always designed to reach students of all levels. Kat's teachings are rooted in the true embodied knowledge that comes from a lifetime of personal experience.

Kat is the host of The Soul Awakening Podcast, is an E-RYT 500, a YA Continued Education Provider, a certified a Reiki Master Teacher, an Advanced Certified Energy Therapist, an Akashic Records Reader, and an experienced teacher's mentor with over a decade of teaching and over 2,000 hours of training. Kat has several beginner to advanced level international online certification courses, including courses on Meditation, Reiki Healing, and the Akashic Records. Additionally, Kat has trained and personally mentored hundreds of teachers collectively at different prestigious yoga and meditation studios and schools in NYC and online. She also guest teaches and lectures at several training programs and international conferences and also speaks at several panel events annually. Kat has been featured on the cover of Yoga Journal, Om Yoga Magazine, NY Yoga + Life Magazine and Natural Awakenings Magazine, as well as in various video and print interviews for Shape magazine, Natural Health Magazine, Manhattan Magazine, and other publications. The Soul Awakening Podcast is available for listening anywhere podcasts are found. For more information about Kat Fowler and her current courses and workshops, visit: www.katfowler.com.

Index